DAVIS COUNTY SC
SCHOOL FOOD SERVICE DEPARTMENT
45 East State Street
Farmington, Utah 84025

LET
THEM
EAT
PROMISES

The
Politics
of
Hunger
in
America

# LET THEM EAT PROMISES

The
Politics
of
Hunger
in
America

By Nick Kotz

*with an introduction by Senator George S. McGovern*

Prentice-Hall, Inc., Englewood Cliffs, New Jersey

*For Jack*

# FOREWORD

HUNGER IS A UNIQUE ISSUE IN CONTEMPORARY
American politics in that it has only been "discovered" in
the late 1960's. Until recently, most Americans assumed
that hunger and malnutrition are the afflictions of Asia
and other faraway places. How could anyone really be
hungry in the world's richest nation—a nation endowed
with an agricultural productivity so vast that it has ac-
cumulated troublesome surpluses? But with mounting
evidence that there are perhaps fifteen million malnourished Americans, the issue of hunger has burst upon the
nation with dramatic force.

Nick Kotz, an unusually perceptive American journalist,
has chronicled this issue in the deeply moving account
which follows. No man is better endowed to describe
"The Politics of Hunger in America" than Mr. Kotz. For
several years, he has placed himself at the center of the

gathering storm swirling around the issues of hunger and malnutrition in affluent America. Now he has skillfully analyzed those issues and given us the tale of political intrigue and struggle associated with them.

A combination of events catapulted hunger into the public spotlight, beginning with the investigation in the Mississippi Delta early in 1967 by Senators Joseph Clark, Robert Kennedy, and their committee colleagues. There followed the brilliant CBS documentary on hunger in America; the hard-hitting study by the Citizens' Board of Inquiry, *Hunger USA;* a highly effective study of the school lunch program, "Their Daily Bread," coordinated by Miss Jean Fairfax; and the creation of the Senate Select Committee on Nutrition and Human Needs, which I have been privileged to serve as chairman.

Hunger is unique as a public issue not only because it is newly recognized but because it exerts a special claim on the conscience of the American people. It is the cutting edge of the problem of poverty. Somehow, we Americans are able to look past the slum housing, the polluted air and water, the bad schools, the excessive population growth, and the chronic unemployment of our poor. But the knowledge that human beings, especially little children, are suffering from hunger profoundly disturbs the American conscience. There is a sense, too, in which it outrages the Puritan ethic to have billions spent to stop food from being grown and finance surplus storage while other Americans languish under the blight of malnutrition.

I saw this same phenomenon operating when I headed President Kennedy's Food for Peace Program in 1961-62. "Foreign Aid" was unpopular and controversial, but feeding the hungry abroad from our overflowing granaries, "Food for Peace," was a highly popular program in the Congress and among the American people.

*viii*

It may be assumed, perhaps, that one of the reasons some men, even some in high positions, have resisted the mounting evidence of widespread malnutrition in the United States stems from these same considerations. To admit the existence of hunger in America is to confess that we have failed in meeting the most sensitive and painful of human needs. To admit the existence of widespread hunger is to cast doubt on the efficacy of our whole system. If we cannot solve the problem of hunger in our society, one wonders if we can resolve any of the great social issues before the nation.

In a fascinating account of the 1968 presidential campaign, three perceptive British journalists concluded that "the most disturbing problem in American politics is . . . the gap between rhetoric and reality." Mr. Kotz sets "the politics of hunger" in a long line of frustrated promises that have separated rhetoric from reality. The Full Employment Act of 1946 promised useful employment to every citizen able and willing to work; yet, millions remain jobless. The Housing Act of 1949 pledged "a decent home in a suitable living environment for every American family"; yet today, six million families exist in miserable hovels across the land. In 1964 the Johnson Administration launched a drive to end poverty in America, but poverty clings stubbornly to the American scene.

Now we have the pledge of the new Nixon Administration to "put an end to hunger in America itself for all time." Is this another bright promise destined to falter on the shoals of inertia, bureaucracy, and rival priorities? This book leaves that question unanswered. "The politics of hunger in America," the author concludes, "is a dismal story of human greed and callousness, and immorality sanctioned and aided by the government of the United

States. But it is also a story that does provide hope that men can change things; that men do care about fulfilling this country's highest ideals, and do care about their fellow human beings."

The account which follows will do much to strengthen the "hope that men can change things."

George McGovern
U.S. Senator, South Dakota
Chairman, Senate Select Committee on
Nutrition and Human Needs

# ACKNOWLEDGMENTS

I first saw the realities of extreme rural poverty through the eyes of my wife, Mary Lynn, on a 1960 trip to her native state of Mississippi. The insights she has given me are not ones about politics, racial conflict, or government programs, but rather the feelings of a sensitive woman on re-encountering the suffering of human beings whom she loves dearly. Working as a newspaper reporter, I saw similar suffering and injustice in Iowa, the golden bread-basket of this nation's prosperity. Returning to Mississippi and other parts of the rural South in 1967 as a Washington correspondent reporting on government programs supposedly designed to alleviate poverty, it seemed to me that the misery was worse than it had been seven years earlier.

This book represents an attempt to tell the story of the discovery of hunger as a national political issue in 1967, and the ensuing struggle both in and out of government to do something about it. The problems of hunger and malnutrition obviously are intertwined with the most perplexing and complicated total problems of poverty and of our domestic society. The hunger issue cannot be isolated, just as one cannot isolate problems of education, jobs, housing, health, and race. This book focuses primarily on the immediate problems of hunger and malnutrition, which seem to me to be the aspects of poverty most susceptible to rational solution, and least excusable in the richest nation in history.

Many people contributed to this book. Foremost, I must thank the poor hungry Americans who, incredibly, still are willing to invite reporters into their homes, who still express faith in the essential goodness of our institutions, who still hope that promises in America will be kept.

Those Americans who have worked to make hunger into a national issue and to end this painful condition have my admiration and appreciation. In particular, I must thank: the late Senator Robert F. Kennedy, Dr. Aaron Altschul, Richard W. Boone, Edgar S. Cahn, Robert B. Choate, former Senator Joseph S. Clark, Clay Cochran, Dr. Robert Coles and his five associates who wrote "Children in Mississippi," Senator Marlow W. Cook, Kenneth L. Dean, Leslie W. Dunbar and members of the Citizen's Board of Inquiry into Hunger and Malnutrition in the United States, Marian Wright Edelman, Peter B. Edelman, Dr. Joseph English, Representative Thomas S. Foley, Jean Fairfax and the Committee on School Lunch Participation, Richard Falknor, Dr. Donald Gatch, Senator Charles E. Goodell, James D. Grant, Fannie Lou Hamer, David Hearne, Senator Ernest F. Hollings, Harry Huge, Senator Jacob K. Javits, Thomas Karter, John R. Kramer, Dr. Charles Upton Lowe, McKinley Martin, Dr. Jean Mayer, Senator George McGovern, Senator Walter F. Mondale, Amzie Moore, Robert Patricelli, William C. Payne, Representative Albert Quie, Duff Reed, S. Stephen Rosenfeld, Dr. Arnold Schaefer, Dr. Aaron Shirley, Kenneth Schlossberg, William C. Smith, Peter Stavrianos, Benton J. Stong, and Kenneth Vallis.

Many officials of the Johnson and Nixon administrations provided valuable information and documents, even when these did not cast them in a favorable light, and I appreciate their honesty and cooperation.

Although this book criticizes the American press for its slowness to report the hunger issue and its failure to understand the Poor People's Campaign, the exceptional reporting of several reporters and their news media accounts in large measure for whatever public understanding and government reforms have been achieved. Among those who covered the story, I owe special thanks to: Sam Adams, Jack Anderson, Mark Arnold, James K. Batten, Dale Bell and the Public Broadcast Laboratory staff who produced "Hunger—American Style," Homer Bigart, William M. Blair, Jerome S. Cahill, Martin Carr and the CBS Television staff who produced "Hunger in America," William T. Chapman, Jo Cullison, Elizabeth Brenner Drew, Eve Edstrom, Paul Good, John A. Hamilton, Richard Harwood, William Hedgepeth, Don Hewitt, Marjorie Hunter, Richard P. Kleeman, Carl P. Leubsdorf, Robert C. Maynard, David M. Mazie, Don Oberdorfer, Lawrence M. O'Rourke, John O'Toole, Carol Oughton, the late Drew Pearson, Judith Randal, Charles and Bonnie Remsburg, Spencer A. Rich, Linda Rockey, Carl Rowan, Daniel Schorr, Burton L. Schorr, Bynum Shaw, Robert Sherrill who wrote the first major story, William Steif, Laurence Stern, Joseph R. L. Sterne, Richard L. Strout, and Calvin Trillin.

Valuable assistance in shaping the manuscript was provided generously by Charles W. Bailey II, Amy Millen, my mother, Tybe Kotz, Elizabeth N. Shiver, Lewis W. Wolfson, and by my fine copy editor, Philip Rosenberg. Sheila Swift typed several versions of the manuscript, and Barbara Ketchum assisted in research. William R. Grose, my editor at Prentice-Hall, provided limitless patience and good judgment. Pat Munroe, Prentice-Hall's Washington representative helped in many ways. Richard L. Wilson, the Washington bureau chief of the Des Moines Register, encouraged me to follow this story and graciously gave me the time to write it. My son, Jack Mitchell Kotz, gave me the priceless qualities of interest, understanding, and much pencil-sharpening.

Finally, my wife, Mary Lynn, was a partner in all phases of writing this book. Her contributions included research, extensive editing, the complete writing of a second draft of the manuscript, and offering endless encouragement.

My hope is that telling this story will result in there being less hunger and malnutrition in America.

Washington, D.C.

# CONTENTS

*This story concerns the politics of hunger in affluent America. It is the story of how some leaders left their air-conditioned sanctuaries, discovered hunger among the poor, and determined to make it into a national issue; of other men who knew about hunger but lied; of still others who learned about hunger but voted for fiscal economy at the expense of the hungry poor.*

# CHAPTER I

# The Discovery of Hunger

HUNGER IN AMERICA WAS CONCEIVED AS A NA-
tional issue in April 1967 by two northern senators in an
alien rural South. On a mission guided by politics, they
came to study poverty programs, but in the small Delta
town of Cleveland, Mississippi, they found more than
they had bargained for.

The United States Senator from New York felt his way
through a dark, windowless shack, fighting nausea at the
strong smell of aging mildew, sickness, and urine. In
the early afternoon shadows, he saw a child sitting on the
floor of a tiny back room. Barely two years old, wearing
only a filthy undershirt, she sat rubbing several grains of
rice round and round on the floor. The senator knelt
beside her.

"Hello . . . Hi . . . Hi, baby . . ." he murmured, touch-
ing her cheeks and her hair as he would his own child's.

As he sat on the dirty floor, he placed his hand gently on the child's swollen stomach. But the little girl sat as if in a trance, her sad eyes turned downward, and rubbed the gritty rice.

For five minutes he tried: talking, caressing, tickling, poking—demanding that the child respond. The baby never looked up.

The senator made his way to the front yard where Annie White, the mother of the listless girl and five other children, stood washing her family's clothes in a zinc tub. She had no money, she was saying to the other senator, couldn't afford to buy food stamps; she was feeding her family only some rice and biscuits made from leftover surplus commodities.

For a few moments Robert F. Kennedy stood alone, controlling his feelings, which were exposed to the press entourage waiting outside the house. Then he whispered to a companion, "I've seen bad things in West Virginia, but I've never seen anything like this anywhere in the United States."

Senators Kennedy of New York and Joseph Clark of Pennsylvania discovered hunger that day, raw hunger imbedded in the worst poverty the black South had known since the Depression of the 1930s. Driving along muddy, forgotten roads, the two senators and their aides stopped at shack after shack to see with their own eyes hungry, diseased children; to hear with their own ears the poor describe their struggle for survival.

The Senate Subcommittee on Employment, Manpower, and Poverty had come to Mississippi to hold hearings, but a tour of Delta homes was not part of the official itinerary. They were taken at the urging of Marian Wright,* a 27-

* Now Mrs. Peter Edelman.

2

year-old civil rights attorney who lived and breathed the problems of the black poor of Mississippi. Miss Wright had testified that people were starving in the cotton-rich Delta, but it was not until she persuaded the two senators to go into the miserable shacks, meet the people, and discover it for themselves that they determined, with deepest conviction, to demand help for the hungry poor.

As a lawyer for the NAACP Legal Defense Fund, Marian Wright had watched the poverty grow more desperate as she grappled with problems of voting rights, welfare rights, and the matter of food itself. This young, black attorney, who grew up in South Carolina and learned law at Yale, had become a catalyst for social reform. Every step of the trip from Washington to the door of Mrs. White's shack had been paved by Marian Wright's advocacy.

When the poverty subcommittee had held Washington hearings the previous month, Republican Senator Jacob Javits of New York called her as he sought unvarnished evaluations of the new poverty programs—truths he feared would not be forthcoming from spokesmen for the Johnson Administration.

As the petite, delicate-featured Marian Wright began testifying, the committee members took notice. Her eloquence is born of deep understanding and compassion, but it was her delivery—rapidly hammering out steel-hard facts in a soft, feminine voice—that caused the bored congressmen to turn in their chairs.

In great detail, she described the suffering of Negro children and adults affected by a Delta area revolution—a revolution produced by the combined effects of mechanized cotton farming, a new minimum wage for farm workers, a huge cutback in cotton planting under the federal subsidy program, and the rising battle for Negro

3

civil rights. Several hundred thousand Negroes were out of work, hungry and unwanted, as mechanization of cotton planting and picking had eliminated the meager jobs on which they had subsisted for generations. And, as a final blow, many counties were switching from a food program in which the poor were given free surplus commodities to a new food stamp program in which stamps cost more than they could possibly pay.

Take the effect of these revolutionary changes on Mississippi Senator James O. Eastland and one of his farm workers, Atley Taylor, for example. The acreage cutback meant federal subsidy payments to the senator of more than $160,000 in 1967, but fewer acres for his laborers to work. Farm mechanization meant that ten tractor drivers had replaced several hundred blacks like Taylor who for years had picked his cotton for $3 per day or less. The $1 per hour * minimum wage meant that it was now cheaper for the senator to spray weed-killing chemicals than to pay the Taylors and others for 30 days of weeding. And finally, the switch in food programs cost the jobless Atley Taylor and his family their free surplus commodities. They had no income—or prospect of any—with which to buy food stamps. The Taylors and thousands of other families often went hungry as Sunflower County's participation in federal food aid dropped from 18,540 persons in the commodity program to 7,856 in food stamps.

Marian Wright's testimony confirmed chairman Clark's judgment that the subcommittee should hold a hearing in the rural South. But, for political reasons, he chose to go to Mississippi rather than to Georgia or Alabama—scenes of similar rural poverty. When a sena-

* Now $1.30.

4

tor prepares to delve into controversial matters, he must consider that no politician appreciates an outsider's exposing problems in his home territory. Although he had always been regarded as a liberal maverick, Clark chose not to offend Georgia's Senate patriarch Richard Russell or Alabama's Lister Hill, chairman of the Senate Labor and Public Welfare Committee, the parent of Clark's poverty subcommittee. He worried less about the good will of Mississippi Senators John Stennis and James Eastland.

Because of these subtle political considerations, Senators Clark and Kennedy, Javits, and George Murphy of California assembled on April 10 in the ballroom of Jackson, Mississippi's crusty old Heidelberg Hotel. The Poverty Subcommittee hearings opened with wrangling about the administration of Head Start programs, and Senator Stennis was there to add his denunciation of the War on Poverty. But Marian Wright was determined to turn their attention to a basic human need.

"People are starving," she testified. "They are starving and those that get the bus fare to go north are trying to go north. There is absolutely nothing for them to do here. There is nowhere to go, and somebody must begin to respond to them. I wish the senators would have a chance to go and just look at the empty cupboards in the Delta and the number of people who are going around begging just to feed their children. Starvation is a major, major problem now."

Miss Wright leveled one of the most damning criticisms one can make of a civilized people, as she said that the withholding of food aid seemed *designed* to drive an unwanted black population out of the state.

Deeply moved and shocked by her testimony and by the words of the poor themselves, Senator Clark sug-

5

gested that the subcommittee members write a joint letter of protest to Agriculture Secretary Orville Freeman. At that point, a conservative member of the subcommittee escalated the politics of hunger.

"If people are starving," said Senator George Murphy, "I don't think the procedure is to go to the Department of Agriculture. I think more drastic means are needed, and I would respectfully suggest that this committee notify the President of the United States that there is an emergency situation, and [to] send investigators and help immediately."

Clark, stunned by Murphy's reaction, sensed that he was about to be upstaged and his Democratic party embarrassed by a conservative Republican. He immediately became far more forceful. His young subcommittee counsel, William C. Smith, hastily drafted a statement expressing Clark's resolve to investigate hunger and carry the issue to President Lyndon Johnson. Ironically, it was former movie actor George Murphy, friend of the California grape grower, who had pushed the liberal Democrats into action on the hunger issue.

Republicans Murphy and Javits returned to Washington the next morning. But Democrats Clark and Kennedy toured the countryside, and thereby informed many Americans about Annie White's baby girl and the thousands like her in Mississippi. For a day, at least, hunger was a minor national issue, principally because Robert Kennedy was news.

Obviously, hunger in affluent America and failure of federal food aid was no secret to the poor, nor to the poverty workers whose pleas for help seemed lost in a political vacuum; nor to the few congressmen like Joseph Resnick of New York, who had found the same hunger in Mississippi 18 months earlier but could get no re-

6

sponse *; nor to the Mississippi poor who had camped across from the White House in early 1966 to demonstrate their desperate plight. But with Robert Kennedy it could be different; with his considerable resources and the public attention always focused on him, he could command a nationwide interest in the problem.

The day after they returned to Washington, Clark and Kennedy went to Agriculture Secretary Orville Freeman to seek emergency help for the hungry of Mississippi. They urgently described to Freeman what they had seen; he seemed sympathetic and before the meeting was over ordered two of his top aides to leave immediately for Mississippi to investigate the food problem. That meeting, in Freeman's expansive office on April 12, 1967, began a Washington battle for food aid reform that is still raging.

Although Kennedy's discovery commanded brief national attention, two citizen forces, unrelated to each other, had already become deeply concerned about hunger in America. Both the Field Foundation and the Citizens' Crusade Against Poverty † were involved in projects to help the hungry poor, and they found impetus in the Kennedy-Clark trip.

Financed by Chicago's Marshall Field department store family, the Field Foundation of New York has long been considered a singularly courageous institution. Where other foundations have supported safe "brick and mortar" projects which ended with a plaque honoring the foundation's gift, Field has risked investing money in causes, including politically unpopular ones,

---

* Resnick, who made a trip to Mississippi to investigate poverty problems, was defeated in a 1968 bid for the Democratic senatorial nomination in New York.

† Now the Center for Community Change.

to help poor people in general, and poor children in particular. Its risk-taking included such activities as giving money to people it could not control and making long-term commitments (another uncommon foundation trait) to such projects as voter education in the South and to a Head Start program the federal government was afraid to finance. The foundation has been sparked in these efforts by Mrs. Marshall Field, by its liberal board members, including such men as Morris Abram, president of Brandeis University, and by its director Leslie W. Dunbar.

A soft-spoken white southerner who grew up in poverty, former college professor Dunbar has devoted his life to helping the black and white poor of his native region. The bespectacled 48-year-old foundation director began his antipoverty efforts with the Southern Regional Council, then moved to the Field Foundation, where he continued his interest in supporting voter education in the South. Thousands of dollars were contributed, on the theory that effective use of the political process is essential to solving problems of discrimination and poverty. (It is projects such as these which prompt southern congressmen to talk about eliminating tax exemptions for foundations.)

Through his deep involvement in Mississippi Head Start projects and contact with leaders like Marian Wright, Leslie Dunbar knew there were hungry black children in Mississippi.

Reading the *New York Times* account of the Kennedy-Clark hunger discovery, the foundation director decided in April 1967 to implement a long-planned trip of his own. From his Park Avenue office Dunbar called one of his board members, Dr. Robert Coles, a Harvard psychiatrist who works devotedly with children of poverty.

8

"Bob, we've been talking about a medical project for the Head Start kids in Mississippi," said Dunbar. "I think it's time to get a team of doctors down there to look at both the medical situation and the food situation."

On Memorial Day weekend, Robert Coles and three other doctors * sponsored by the Field Foundation went to Mississippi to examine children at Head Start centers throughout the state. As they traveled through seven counties in the rich, flat Delta, and in the adjoining hill country, their indignation mounted. The four doctors, all veterans of missions into poverty-stricken areas, were appalled at the condition of the Negro children they saw.

The stark details of horribly diseased children, suffering from severe dietary deficiencies and hopelessly inadequate diets, were vividly captured in a report they presented in early June, on "Children in Mississippi."

". . . We saw children being fed communally—that is by neighbors who give scraps of food to children whose own parents have nothing to give them. Not only are these children receiving no food from the government, they are also getting no medical attention whatsoever. They are out of sight and ignored. They are living under such primitive conditions that we found it hard to believe we were examining American children of the twentieth century!"

By the time the Field Foundation doctors left Mississippi, each was outraged that children should suffer such pain and neglect in the midst of affluent America. Small wonder that the Negro infant mortality rate in Mississippi

---

* The other doctors were Dr. Joseph Brenner, of Massachusetts Institute of Technology, Dr. Alan Merman of Yale University Medical School, and Dr. Raymond Wheeler, from North Carolina. Dr. Cyril Walwyn of Mississippi joined the doctors in Mississippi. Dr. Milton Senn of Yale joined in their report.

was double that of whites and rising, while the white rate was falling. They called for immediate emergency medical treatment and food aid.

With images of Mississippi children still seared in their minds, the doctors flew to Washington on June 16 to demand action from the highest government officials responsible for food, medical, and poverty aid. They began the day confident that such liberals as Agriculture Secretary Orville Freeman, Health, Education, and Welfare Secretary John Gardner, and Office of Economic Opportunity Director Sargent Shriver would respond with emergency help. By the end of the morning, the four doctors were bitterly disillusioned. Freeman talked about restrictions placed on him by the power of southern conservatives in Congress, and HEW officials talked about political limitations on activities of the Public Health Service.

The dejected physicians trudged on to Capitol Hill, where they told their stories again. But this time there was a response. As luncheon guests of Senators Kennedy and Clark, the doctors described the comments of Freeman and another Department of Agriculture official who chided the doctors for stirring up southern conservatives in Congress. Bob Kennedy replied: "You don't have to take that. This is the beginning, not the end. You don't have to be discouraged."

Kennedy and Clark also had met with Freeman, and despite a dozen requests for emergency aid, they had drawn no positive response. The two senators whispered briefly with each other, and then Clark told the doctors: "We're going to hold more hearings!" The senators pulled out their calendars and set a date in July for the politics of hunger to receive a congressional forum in Washington. For the first time, federal food programs would be examined on Capitol Hill outside the confines of the agriculture committees.

While the senators prepared for Congressional hearings, a citizen group located in a basement office 20 blocks from the Capitol was also considering how to focus attention on the hunger problem.

The Citizens' Crusade Against Poverty had been created in 1965 as liberal support for poverty legislation. Its chief backers—Walter Reuther and his United Auto Workers, the National Council of Churches, the United Presbyterian Church, and the Ford Foundation—conceived of the Crusade as a force to bring together all elements of the liberal community in much the same way that the Leadership Council on Civil Rights had joined liberal groups to champion major civil rights legislation.* But times were changing; as the civil rights revolution began to demand "freedom now," the liberals began to bicker over the proper pace for social reform.

Under the leadership of its executive director Richard W. Boone, the Citizens' Crusade quickly allied itself with black, Mexican-American, and white poverty groups who sought to run their own programs. Because of Boone's interest, the Citizens' Crusade boldly helped poor people develop their own leadership. The Crusade was active in the grapefields of Delano, California, in the ghettoes of Watts and East Los Angeles, in the Woodlawn section of Chicago, and in the rural Mississippi Delta.

With his crew cut and clean good looks, the 42-year-old Boone looks more like a Marine major than a major social reformer. His quiet manner and his dislike of publicity hide the enormous influence he has exercised on national

* An informal coalition of civil rights, religious, labor, and other organizations whose leaders worked in tandem to lobby for civil rights legislation.

social problems. He originated vital antipoverty concepts and projects, such as the principle of "maximum feasible participation by the poor," the Vista Volunteers, Upward Bound, the Foster Grandparents program,* and projects to give American Indians a voice in their own affairs. After a career as police juvenile officer, job training specialist with incorrigible youths, Ford Foundation executive, and designer of federal antipoverty programs, Boone had decided that poor people's own ideas could not be any worse than those of the experts who had failed to solve the problem of poverty.

He was infuriated by the vast discrepancy between the promise of the Great Society and the actual performance of its programs. When the energetic Marian Wright and other members of his rural affairs committee had told him about the desperate situation in Mississippi and the failure of federal food aid programs, Boone immediately saw a role for the Citizens' Crusade. Support for antipoverty efforts had grown hopelessly diffuse, he felt, and a new issue could provide a dramatic focus on poverty. "What could be more basic than hunger?" he asked.

By coincidence, on the same day that Kennedy and Clark discovered Annie White's child in Mississippi, Boone had presented the cause of hunger to his board of directors, who gave him the go-ahead. Two months later, while Kennedy and Clark were setting up their hearings, Boone sat in his office and listened as his associate Robert B. Choate poured out facts and figures that gave a greatly expanded picture of the hunger problem.

"It's a national scandal," Choate reported. "There must be millions of people going hungry all over America." A Boston aristocrat with a strong streak of New England

* All three are popular, successful OEO programs.

12

moral outrage at social injustice, Choate had trained as an engineer but devoted most of his life to breaking new ground in the poverty fight. Using U.S. Census and other government data, he plotted out, state by state and county by county, pertinent statistics on 29 million poor Americans. Most graphically, his statistics disclosed a persistent relationship throughout the country between poverty and high infant mortality rates and the lack of adequate government food and welfare aid. Where poverty was greatest, so was infant mortality, and food and welfare benefits were lowest.

Armed with Choate's new profile of poverty, Boone determined to form a special "Citizens' Board of Inquiry into Hunger and Malnutrition in the United States" with the objective of focusing national attention on the problem of hunger.

By mid-June 1967, efforts of the three independent forces began to merge and a new antihunger lobby came into being. Dr. Coles and the other Field Foundation-sponsored doctors prepared to testify at Clark's Senate hearing; and the first person Boone called as he decided how best to form the Board of Inquiry was Leslie Dunbar. It was a natural action because Boone and Dunbar had worked together on southern poverty problems and they both felt that concentration on long-term planning was irrelevant when children were suffering terrible deprivation.

"How can anyone think of other things until we deal with hunger?" Dunbar told Boone, agreeing to commit the financial support of the Field Foundation and to serve as co-chairman of the Board of Inquiry.*

In July the 25-member Citizens' Board of Inquiry met

---

* The other co-chairman was Dr. Benjamin Mays, president of Morehouse College, Atlanta, Georgia.

in New York to map out the first full-scale examination of government food aid programs. Richard Boone and co-chairman Leslie Dunbar had selected respected figures from medicine, law, universities, foundations, social action groups, organized labor, and religion.* (The food industry, whose top executives showed little interest in serving, was notable in its absence.) The Board quickly moved into action, so that scarcely three months after the visit to Annie White's shack, the resources and man-

* The other members were: Harry S. Ashmore, author, Center for the Study of Democratic Institutions; James P. Carter, M. D., Pediatrician, Division of Nutrition, Vanderbilt University; Rt. Rev. Daniel Corrigan, Director, Home Department, Executive Council of the Episcopal Church; Norman Dorsen, Professor of Law, Director, Arthur Garfield Hays Civil Liberties program, New York University School of Law; Rashi Fein, senior staff member for economic studies, the Brookings Institution; M. Alfred Haynes, M. D., Associate Professor of International Health, Johns Hopkins School of Hygiene and Public Health; Vivian W. Henderson, President, Clark College; Fay Bennett, Executive Secretary, National Sharecroppers Fund; Msgr. Lawrence J. Corcoran, Secretary, National Conference of Catholic Charities; Vine Deloria, Executive Director, National Congress of American Indians; George Esser, Executive Director, the North Carolina Fund; Stanley N. Gershoff, Associate Professor of Nutrition, Harvard University School of Public Health; Ralph Helstein, President, United Packinghouse, Food, and Allied Workers; Dolores Huerta, Secretary, United Farm Workers Organizing Committee; Harry Huge, attorney, Arnold & Porter, Washington, D. C.; Rabbi Robert Kahn, Congregation Emanu-El, Houston, Texas; James O'Connor, President, American Freedom from Hunger Foundation; Gilbert Ortiz, M. D., Chairman of ASPIRA, the Bronx, N.Y.; Edward Sparer, Professor of Law, Yale University; Walter Mitchell, President, International Chemical Workers Union; Milton Ogle, Executive Director, Appalachian Volunteers; Phillip Sorenson, Executive Director, Irwin-Sweeney-Miller Foundation; Raymond Wheeler, M. D., Charlotte Medical Clinic, Charlotte, N. C.

14

power to investigate hunger and malnutrition had been organized and were moving into poverty pockets throughout the nation.

The initial actions by the Senate Poverty Subcommittee, the Citizens' Crusade, and the Field Foundation took place almost simultaneously, and in the eyes of some it looked like a Kennedy political plot. To Representative Jamie Whitten, a Mississippi Democrat and the powerful chairman of the House Appropriations Subcommittee on Agriculture, it was both a Kennedy plot and a liberal ploy to gain Negro votes by maligning the South.

Neither conjecture was true, although everyone involved knew each other, most were Kennedy supporters, and their joining forces was no accident. The way they came to focus on the essential problem of hunger which was hidden beneath the veneer of the War on Poverty is the story of a new kind of politics in action.

Poverty pioneers Marian Wright, Dunbar, Boone, and Coles had bonds of shared experience and common philosophy. All believed that the poor must be given a major voice in decisions about programs affecting their lives. All realized that government welfare institutions were functioning poorly, with a ponderous federal bureaucracy tied ineffectually to state and local governments in a weblike system which always seemed to neglect the poor. All knew that the only real test of antipoverty programs is whether they actually help the hard-core poor. The four had been brought together once before and now were led to the hunger issue by their common support for an embattled multi-county Head Start program that had tested the morality of President Lyndon B. Johnson's poverty war.

For the poor Negroes who received the federal funds and directed the Child Development Group of Mississippi, Head Start had been a first experience in self-government. Aside from the benefits to children, who would now see a doctor, a carrot, or a crayon for the first time, the Head Start centers also brought together their parents, who drew strength from each other as they traded stories about food, welfare, and job problems. The efforts were embryonic and weak, often disorganized and inefficient, but poor blacks in Mississippi were starting to develop a voice.

Participation by the poor in government programs would be a radical policy in the North (where even liberal congressmen feared the poor would organize to defeat the established leadership), but in Mississippi it was downright revolutionary. The segregationist political power structure of the South, led by Senators Eastland and Stennis, tried for more than two years to destroy the Head Start program. Boone, Dunbar, and Marian Wright lobbied hard to keep the Johnson Administration from killing Mississippi's Head Start centers and helped on the local scene with leadership training, funds, and legal counsel. Because of their efforts, the Head Start program survived.

Working closely with poor people, these leaders were well aware of hunger in Mississippi, but Robert Kennedy was undergoing a new experience and beginning a new kind of politics. Kennedy had not helped out in the Head Start fight. He had been initially unsympathetic and uncomprehending in those days. He had never heard of the new breed of Mississippi Negro leaders like Fannie Lou Hamer,* but he did know and respect the more traditional Negro and white leaders who offered a rival, compromise Mississippi Head Start program.

---

* Mrs. Hamer first gained national attention when she eloquently pleaded the case for Negro political rights at the 1964 Democratic National Convention.

Kennedy brought to Mississippi a theory about poverty hearings—a theory which would quickly lead to his own education and join him with the other food aid reformers. Convinced that congressional hearings should be used as a forum to expose the problems of poverty, he believed that the poor themselves made the best witnesses, that little was accomplished in hearings devoted to the opinions of bureaucrats and local politicians. When the Poverty Subcommittee made the first stop of its tour at a job training center in Greenville, Mississippi, the center's director infuriated Kennedy by his inability to answer a single question—even a question as vital as how many of the trainees had gotten jobs. From that moment on, Kennedy took command of the tour—and of subsequent tours—demanding that the subcommittee concentrate on hearing the poor and visiting them where they lived.

In fact, Robert Kennedy himself was undergoing a rapid political evolution in which the Mississippi experience played an important role. Urged on by young aides Peter Edelman and Adam Walinsky, Kennedy came more and more to identify with the aspirations of the forgotten Americans. He went to Indian reservations, to Appalachia, and into New York City ghettoes, and gradually he came to *feel* poverty, to feel pain for the poor. Politically, the young senator probably was doing the right thing for himself, going toward the groups naturally attracted to him. It may have been good politics for Kennedy to get to the left of the Johnson Administration, and it suited his style to visit and be photographed with his constituency of forgotten and oppressed Americans. But Robert Kennedy also was learning, and he was an existential politician who learned by experiencing emotions. As a sensitive observer, he was penetrating the deceptive facade of legislative purposes and bureaucratic statistics when he went into shacks like the ones in Cleveland, Mississippi.

*17*

All these experiences eventually merged in a protest about the quality of American society, in a litany for the forgotten poor: "There are millions of Americans living in hidden places whose faces and names we never know. But I have seen the children starving in Mississippi, idling their lives away in the urban ghetto, living without hope or future amid the despair of Indian reservations. These conditions will change, those children will live, only if we dissent."

During the 35 years since Franklin Roosevelt's New Deal began shaping the welfare state, the hard-core poor had been systematically excluded from the decision-making process and from most of the social welfare benefits which made life easier for other Americans. The older liberal leaders, self-satisfied with their legislative record and their creation of massive federal bureaucracies, either did not hear or could not understand the new language of the 1960s. To them, voices of the poor sounded shrilly unpleasant, "radical," and certainly ungrateful and unappreciative of liberal accomplishments.

When hunger reached a crisis stage in Mississippi, Kennedy and his new allies were attuned to those voices. The food aid reformers listened, and began their campaign for food with a new politics of hunger. Supporting the public figures was a dedicated team of quiet, intelligent, concerned men who guided these independent forces throughout the hunger crusade. Kennedy legislative assistant Peter Edelman, Poverty Subcommittee Counsel William C. Smith, and Minority Counsel Robert Patricelli worked as a unit, coordinating legislative and administrative efforts with the citizen participation of Richard Boone, Robert Choate, and Leslie Dunbar. This was the new cast of characters, who operated deftly behind the scenes, eagerly supporting the Senate hearings and the

Citizens' Board of Inquiry into Hunger and Malnutrition.

Guided by an able professional staff, the Citizens' Board of Inquiry began a Washington-based survey of all data available on malnutrition and government food aid programs. Within weeks key staff members Edgar Cahn and Stephen Rosenfeld gathered enough evidence to see that for years individual doctors had been diagnosing malnutrition problems in poverty groups of the population—yet no one had called for corrective action or seen the pattern as a national problem.

At the same time, Citizens' Board of Inquiry teams went into the ghettoes of Boston and New York, the Indian reservations of South Dakota and Arizona, the rural white slums of Appalachia and rural black slums of South Carolina, the migrant camps of Florida, and the dismal Mexican-American *barrios* of San Antonio. The Board of Inquiry, in effect, was performing a function that Congress had long neglected. Its field trips and public hearings followed the format of congressional investigations and hearings, which are used both to gather facts and to focus public attention on an issue. As the Board moved from state to state, stories of the witnesses followed a familiar pattern. Poor people said they were hungry and were not being helped by government food programs. Local doctors said poor children in their areas suffered from malnutrition. Poverty workers described local institutions that resisted any efforts to alleviate the misery of the poor.

As the Board members investigated, held hearings, and examined children, they confirmed that hunger and malnutrition were not confined to Mississippi.

Hunger was a scar across an affluent nation.

# CHAPTER II

# Out of Sight and Ignored

IN THIS COUNTRY, THOUSANDS OF YOUNG CHILDREN feel pain. Some do not call it "hunger" because they have never known the feeling of a full stomach. Countless Americans are physically and mentally maimed for life, their entire destiny and contribution to society sharply limited by what they eat in the first four years of life or even by what their mothers ate during pregnancy. Hungry children cannot concentrate and do not learn at school; they develop lifetime attitudes about a hostile world. Malnourished men, already handicapped by limited education, are too listless to work. Modern science now has demonstrated clearly that the effects of malnutrition are far more significant than was ever imagined. We are now beginning to learn the costs of hunger—both to our national economy and to the individuals who suffer its effects.

Yet, after hunger and malnutrition among some ten million Americans became a clear political issue, South Carolina's Strom Thurmond and likeminded allies in the United States Senate almost succeeded in curbing a national study of the problem. "There has been hunger since the time of Jesus Christ and there always will be," stated Thurmond.

No one could argue with the first part of the senator's statement. The problem of hunger has been part of the human condition since the beginning, and various solutions, over the centuries, have been integral to the progress of civilization. Hunger has eliminated entire cultures from this planet, has changed the course of history for others. Little more than a hundred years ago, for example, a potato famine in Ireland brought scores of Irish to this country. Other severe food shortages contributed to the waves of immigrants seeking food and freedom in a nation that was rich in both. As we approach the twenty-first century, science has advanced to the point where men have traveled to the moon and returned safely, yet, two-thirds of this world's people still suffer from malnutrition. Entire populations are stunted in physical development because they lack adequate diets. In America, however, the problems of hunger are not even remotely the same as those faced by underdeveloped nations where the population increase is outpacing ancient, outmoded agricultural methods, where the capacity to feed everyone does not exist.

This new American tragedy is that hunger and malnutrition, excruciating human misery and disease, should exist for millions—in the richest nation with the highest individual standard of living known to mankind. This is not the America of frozen colonial winters and men chewing on leather; of American soldiers scavenging for food as they fought their neighbors over questions of Union; of apple-selling Depression days when the poor died quietly and unknown while the very rich died in spectacular leaps from tall buildings that had been constructed of paper. This is the story of hunger in the America of the $900 billion gross national product, of the $200 billion federal budget, of 1.2 cars and 1.3 television sets per family, of eight million pleasure boats, of block-long supermarkets with entire meals frozen to be prepared instantly in automated kitchens. This is the America that pays farmers $3 billion annually not to plant food because it has developed an ingenious ability to produce far more than paying customers can eat, the America that spends millions on dieting because the affluent consumer can afford to eat too well. For the first time, this is the America fully equipped with the ability, the technology, and the wealth to fulfill its most sacred promises—life, liberty, and the pursuit of happiness.

Yet this nation in the late 1960s looked hunger in the eyes but could not see it, glimpsed the truth about hunger but called only for more study of the problem, discounted hunger as a result of either laziness or ignorance, and finally—even after it reluctantly accepted the problem— could not arrange its national priorities to feed more than a fraction of the malnourished and hungry poor in 1970.

The nation should not have needed a survey to know that many millions of Americans suffer from inadequate nutrition, not because they are ignorant about proper diet, but because they are poor. More than one million Americans live in families with no income at all. Another five million Americans have less total income than the amount the Agriculture Department estimates is needed to maintain a barely minimum diet. Another nine million have such low income that maintaining an adequate diet would require spending from 50 to 100 percent of their meager funds on food alone. How can any of these 15 million poor Americans afford proper nutrition?

The answer is that millions cannot, and the government now is admitting it.

The federal government's own definition of poverty—income less than three times the cost of a minimum diet—should have offered strong clues about hunger. A family of four is considered poor if it has less than $3,600 a year, or three times the $1,200 income needed for food.*

The National Food Consumption Survey reported in 1955 that almost 25 percent of American families in poverty had diets seriously lacking in essential nutrients, and by 1965 the number had risen to 36 percent. The gap between the affluent and the very poor in America had widened, with the poor increasingly incapable of keeping up with a rising cost of survival.

When hunger in America exploded into a national concern in the late 1960's, many Americans were incredulous, wondering whether it really existed and how it suddenly became a political issue. Among the curious was President Richard Nixon, who questioned his highest White House advisers.

"Hunger would have been worse in the late 1950s, and we never heard about it then," the President told members of his Cabinet.

During the recession of the late 1950s, hunger *had* been a problem, raising questions about woefully insufficient food aid to the jobless, but it never gained momentum as a political issue. During the 1960 Presidential campaign, John F. Kennedy had said that 17 million Americans go to bed hungry at night, but pressured by opponent Nixon

---

* Prior to 1965 the figures were $3,000 a year, or three times the $1,000 income needed for food.

to clarify that statement, Kennedy explained that he was quoting statistics on potential malnutrition.

Moved by the poverty he saw during the West Virginia primary, President Kennedy, on his first day in office, doubled the existing commodity aid program, and during the following years the quantity of food aid was expanded greatly. Compared to existing programs, these reforms were impressive; compared to the need, they were minimal. The fact that millions of Americans had too little to eat still made no strong impression on government or the public, and there still was no national commitment.

How could mass hunger among the American poor be ignored for so long? Why did the food aid reformers succeed in drawing attention to the subject in 1967 when others before them had failed?

To answer these questions, to follow the hunger story to its source, trace the history of certain American institutions. Travel to the plantation country of the Deep South to learn how its peculiar political, social, and economic institutions really operate for the cotton planter and for the black cotton worker; visit the company coal town in Appalachia to glimpse the effect of its institutions on the lives of miner, management, and absentee owner; walk in the rich fruit and vegetable valleys of Texas and California to see how life is shaped for the grower and for the Mexican-American picker. Follow agricultural laborers along the migrant stream to see how they fit into the institutions of Connecticut at tobacco picking time and of Iowa during the vegetable harvest; study the American Indian from Colonial days to his present home on a United States government reservation. And finally, to understand fully how poor people fit into a *new* set of American institutions, go along with all these forgotten

Americans as they move into the bulging urban ghettoes.

The trip is an illuminating one. Many Americans, particularly the brightest, most concerned young men and women, traveled this road in the 1960s—examining the myths of our institutions, looking at how they really operate, stripping away the illusions. They discovered that the apparatus of the state, including federal food programs, was used to keep rural Americans from obtaining social, political, or economic equality. They found out, for example, how federal food aid really worked in the cotton belt and the crop-rich southwestern valleys.

Surplus commodities—barely enough to survive on—were distributed in the winter when there was no work on Senator Eastland's Mississippi plantation or on the huge Texas ranches. In the spring, when the $3-a-day planting jobs opened up, the food aid ended. The federal government eased the planter's responsibility by keeping his workers alive during the winter, then permitted counties to withdraw that meager support during planting season—forcing the workers to accept near-starvation wages in order to survive. Even those wages vanished when the rural serfs, slowly replaced by coal-digging cotton-picking, and fruit-plucking machines, had outlived their usefulness to the planter. They fled to the cities where a new kind of brutalization took place for men ill-educated and ill-equipped to earn a living there. Thus the United States government worked hand in hand with the most feudal systems of agricultural peonage.

As the Poverty Subcommittee and Citizens' Board of Inquiry traveled the nation, they saw countless examples of food and welfare benefits withheld or granted to suit the needs of local institutions. Food and welfare aid, in minimal amounts, were available for the docile poor who "stayed in line," but these benefits could be withheld from anyone who challenged or threatened the institutions by demanding full participation in society. In Greenwood, Mississippi, food aid benefits were cut off to punish Negroes leading a voter registration drive. In company coal towns of Kentucky, mothers who petitioned that the schools supply their children school lunches found that their schools responded by cutting their children out of the Neighborhood Youth Corps program. Indians in Oklahoma and Mexican-Americans in northern New Mexico learned that new poverty aid went only to those who blindly accepted corrupt local leadership.

Food aid programs in agricultural regions throughout the nation were turned on or off to suit the convenience and labor needs of the growers and planters. Coal companies in Appalachia, cotton planters in the Deep South, and vegetable-fruit growers in the Southwest all tried to keep their cheap labor in virtual bonded indebtedness by advancing them survival funds which they could never repay. The U. S. Department of Labor cooperated fully in the system of migrant labor, by which human beings are shipped and housed like cattle. In a more traditional kind of politics, surplus commodities were distributed in Des Moines and Chicago at the whim of the party bosses. The relationship between the poor and such institutions as local government, business, agriculture, or influential community organizations rarely was examined or understood.

Until the mid-1960s affluent America had never looked closely at the intimate details of extreme poverty. Entire groups of human beings were seen only dimly on the American landscape, as millions of Negroes, Mexican-Americans, Indians, Anglo-Saxon Appalachians, and scattered white men everywhere struggled with problems of poverty that the rest of the country did not comprehend.

The Irish did it, the Italians did it, the Jews did it, we said, and anyone else can succeed in this country, if he works hard enough. We assumed that the poor stayed that way because they wanted to—that they were too lazy and ignorant to lift themselves out of the mire. We never paused to reflect that picking cotton in Mississippi or fruit in California or digging coal in Kentucky are man-breaking jobs not designed for the lazy. We never looked closely enough to see the patterns of poverty, to feel the human tragedy in the lives of the hungry. Most of all, we never thought seriously about why entire groups of Americans were poor. A thorough examination would have challenged some of our notions about our institutions and about our generosity as Americans.

Throughout our history, certain of our citizens have been systematically and legally excluded from the economic and social benefits which are provided to make life better for middle and upper America. The rural black and brown and white Americans whose sweat produced the cotton and the vegetables were the last to receive any of the legislative benefits of child labor regulations, minimum wage laws, unemployment compensation, collective bargaining rights, and social security. Many of these rights are still denied them today. Add to this the oppressive racial and ethnic discrimination that has been sanctioned throughout our history and, in the case of the American Indian, has been government-administered right down to 1969, when babies are dying from lack of food on Navajo reservations. The nation's concept of these "other Americans" was an abstract, distant one at best and never extended as far as an examination of diet and medical health. Even when the entire nation was stricken with the Depression of the 1930s, America responded mainly to meet the temporary economic needs of its middle class.

27

From the 1950s onward the civil rights movement drew increasing attention to the life of the black poor in the South. As the more obvious legal rights were won—at least on paper—the movement turned to the basic conditions of life throughout this country; and the War on Poverty, with its massive failures and overpromised programs, contributed to our learning process. But billion-dollar programs do not automatically solve problems of poverty, and the poor continued to complain, as riots swept the streets.

Throughout the 1960s, the nation expected instant success from its antipoverty efforts. If children continued to drop out of school despite Head Start, if job training courses did not produce instant mechanics, if the poor failed to hold jobs provided them by the magnanimity of private industry, then critics assumed this was proof of their conclusions about the worthlessness of the poor, about their laziness and indifference. It was only after the programs were well under way that the human victims of poverty finally came into view, and the program planners began to realize that generations-rooted poverty does not give way to simple solutions—especially when it is promoted and still supported by the basic local institutions.

A better school may help a child, but not if the child is sick, hungry, and sleepless from a night spent in the turbulent environment of overcrowded housing. A man may desire eagerly to participate in a job training program, but will fail if he lacks basic educational skills or the energy needed to perform the job. Job training will lead only to disillusionment if there is not a job available at the end of the course. If men still suffer and are not helped, it makes little difference that the government pours billions into programs.

The War on Poverty at least was a beginning. Out of the civil rights movement came dignity and self-determination. The Economic Opportunity Act, in its Community Action Program, tried to carry forward these all-American attitudes with a requirement of "maximum feasible participation of the poor"—a concept which met with resistance from political bosses in the cities, segregationist politicians in the South, self-righteous liberals, and well-entrenched philanthropic leaders. For whatever their reasons, most leaders of the established institutions firmly opposed giving the poor a real voice in determining their own future.

But there were important exceptions to this pattern of resistance, and the exceptions included other influential American institutions. Harvard University gave Dr. Robert Coles the freedom to roam the country and help the distressed; the Midwest department store fortune of the Marshall Field family backed Leslie Dunbar's commitment to raising Negro political power in the South; Walter Reuther committed the strength of his labor union to Richard Boone's efforts to develop indigenous leadership in the slums; the prestige and money of the NAACP Legal Defense Fund supported the energetic work of a young lawyer named Marian Wright. Finally, Robert Kennedy, assisted by the able Bill Smith and Peter Edelman, was buttressed by the power of the U.S. Senate, even though other powerful senators opposed his campaign. Each of these individuals worked within the framework of established American society, even as they dissented so that "these conditions will change, those children will live." Demonstrating intelligence, compassion, and courage in initiating the crusade against hunger, each saw the need for change and acted on it.

In the past, poor people spoke, if at all, to the government or the public only through welfare workers, precinct leaders, or plantation bosses. Purposefully or inadvertently, the story was lost in translation. But with new channels open to them, the poor could give vivid accounts of exploitation, discrimination, faulty government programs. They talked about the problems of poverty in terms of inadequate housing and clothing, of missing medical care, and of hostile or indifferent government officials. Now for the first time the poor began to speak for themselves in a voice louder than a whisper.

The voice said, "We are hungry."

# CHAPTER III

# The Cost to America

THE BABY WAS SICK, BUT THE YOUNG PUBLIC
Health Service doctor could not find the cause. At 18
months, the infant's weight was a normal 21 pounds, yet
her hands and feet were swollen, and she cried pitifully
on the examining table.

"She cries all the time," her mother reported.

"What does she eat?" asked the doctor.

"Tea, soda water, and beans," the woman replied.

"How about milk?"

"No," the Navajo Indian mother answered, "We haven't
had milk in a long time, and no meat, either."

In Tuba City, Arizona, Dr. Charles B. Wolf made a
startling diagnosis. The infant suffered from "kwashiorkor," a disease caused by severe protein deficiency, and
characterized by a distended belly, bulging eyes, loss of
hair, and, if untreated, eventual death. The illness, known

as the "starvation disease," is widespread among the most primitive nations of the world, but it rarely had been reported in 20th-century America. During the next few months, Dr. Wolf discovered two more cases of kwashiorkor and countless cases of malnutrition, including marasmus (severe calorie malnutrition).

That was in 1961. Dr. Wolf published his findings and attempted to improve the nutrition of the Navajos who live on the vast reservation that spreads across four southwestern states. The young physician left Tuba City confident that authorities would respond to his reports.

Eight years later, Dr. Jean VanDusen, a physician at the same Public Health Service hospital told Congress that in 1969 she had treated 44 cases of kwashiorkor and marasmus among Indians on the reservation. For the Navajos, starvation is a continuing fact of life.

Although for years a few individual physicians and scientists such as Dr. Wolf had been diagnosing extensive malnutrition among poor Americans and warning of its consequences, no one had drawn the evidence together and read its devastating patterns. Little was known about the nutritional status of the poor—or the rich—in the United States. Neither government nor private medicine had studied the subject extensively or attempted to cope with the problem. The fact of continued neglect, as among the Navajos, was persistently ignored by authorities until the 1960s, when the poor began to speak and the concerned to listen. Only then, in a political forum, did the country begin to examine the consequences of hunger in the United States.

The total cost of hunger in America is incalculable. It limits the potential of this entire nation. It diminishes and indeed makes a mockery of America's promise and

32

of its most noble aspirations. Part of the cost can be measured in economic terms. But it is in terms of the ability of a child to function at school and to respond to his widening world, in terms of a man's ability to work and to respect the society in which he lives that hunger becomes a national tragedy. Finally, the cost of hunger may be measured in terms of human life itself.

In 1969 this abundant United States ranks 27th among nations of the world in life expectancy for men and 15th for women. The infant mortality rate in the United States is higher than that in 14 other countries, including all of western Europe, and in America's ghettoes and rural slums the death rate for black infants is actually increasing. An infant born to poor parents in the United States is twice as likely as his middle-class counterpart to die before reaching his first birthday, and, should he survive the first year of his life, his chance of reaching the age of 35 is four times less than that of the average American. Many factors in the syndrome of poverty contribute to this mortality rate (which for babies can be ten times higher in a poor slum than a rich suburb), but experts point to malnutrition as a key cause. After treating increasing numbers of inadequately fed ghetto infants in his hospital, a Baltimore physician said:

"We pay so much attention to traffic deaths; every day the newspapers tell us how to drive carefully—and yet, if the infant mortality rate was on a par with modern European countries, 50,000 children would not die unnecessarily in this nation each year."

The doctor's numbers may be low. An estimated 148,000 births—most of them among the poor—go unreported, and deaths among these children would not be counted.

Is society blameless in these deaths? As some men

33

studied government food programs that did not feed the hungry, a moral question confronted the American conscience.

Whispers of "planned starvation" emerged from the economic crisis of 1967, after huge cotton production cutbacks and highly automated farm machinery left the Deep South with thousands of no-longer-needed, unemployed blacks—who finally had the vote and the collective will to be treated as men. "It seems you either have to starve or go to Chicago," is the way Negro leader Amzie Moore described the change in Mississippi food programs, a change that is part of the politics of hunger. Whether by neglect or plan, the decisions of white supremacist leaders in the South, supported by the U. S. Department of Agriculture, drove hordes of the destitute into the choked ghettoes of the North, where, unskilled and uneducated, they continued to go hungry.

Our northern liberal consciences should not presume that neglect had been confined to the Deep South, any more than that the deadly kwashiorkor and marasmus were confined to Biafra. Aside from the kwashiorkor found on the Navajo reservation, the National Nutrition Survey in 1969 uncovered 7 cases of the starvation disease among the first 12,000 poor examined.

The painful reality of hunger and malnutrition can be discovered by anyone who journeys to where the "other Americans" live. Most of us do not make that trip, even if it is only a few blocks, and perhaps nontravelers are blinded by a confusion of terms. Many Americans, including county health officials and congressmen, have denied the existence of serious food problems because they associate hunger only with India-style famine—emaciated people dropping like flies in the streets. Of course, if they looked in the right places, they would find cases of starvation: small children with wasted bodies and empty bellies dying from hunger in Arizona, in South Carolina, in the slums of New York City. For most of the 10 to 15 million who suffer from hunger in this country, the effects are more insidious. The ravages of malnutrition go on within the human body, and the body adjusts to it, sacrificing vital brain and body growth and energy.

Much confusion surrounds the words "hunger," "malnutrition," "undernutrition," and "starvation." The terms were used interchangeably—both by physicians and by a general public unaccustomed to thinking about such problems, much less applying those words to this country. In this book, the terms are used as defined by the Senate Select Committee on Nutrition and Human Needs:

"Hunger" is the subjective feeling that results from an individual's lack of food at a particular point of time. However, the term is also used interchangeably with "undernutrition" and "malnutrition" to describe general and prolonged or chronic nutritional deprivation; an impairment or risk of impairment to mental or physical health resulting from a failure to meet dietary requirements; a continued lack of food resulting in periods of prolonged subjective feelings of hunger.

"Malnutrition" is an impairment or risk of impairment to mental or physical health resulting from the failure to meet the total nutrient requirements of an individual.

"Undernutrition" is the consumption of an insufficient quantity of food or of one or more of the essential nutrients.

"Starvation" is the state of advanced undernutrition, the effect of which is wastage of body tissue and ultimate death.

When the six doctors sponsored by the Field Foundation reported on the lack of food in Mississippi in 1967, they provoked an angry debate in which the state's doctors agreed there could be "malnutrition" and possibly some "hunger," but certainly no "starvation." Dr. Raymond Wheeler, one of the doctors who visited Mississippi, tried to explain to the United States Senate that the terms used are far less important than is an understanding of the consequences of inadequate nutrition: "I would say that these adults and children . . . are, in many cases sick, in pain, hungry, and starving—whether one uses the word in a scientific or a humanitarian sense. Why must we quibble about the quantitative effects of food deprivation on the body, or how rapidly one dies because of hunger?

"When a child is weak and apathetic because of anemia," he continued, "stunted in growth, subject to disease which can be fatal because of inadequate body resistance, doomed to permanent mental impairment—all as a result of inadequate food—that child is starving. He will live less fully and die more quickly because he does not have enough to eat."

A "morbid chain" caused by poverty wreaks permanent damage to thousands of young Americans, scientists from the National Institutes of Health reported to the Senate:[*]

Poverty means improperly fed pregnant women . . .

Which means ill-fed fetuses in their wombs . . .

Fetuses which fail to synthesize proteins and brain cells at normal rates . . .

Which means a high rate of mortality among infants . . .

And further lack of brain and body growth during the crucial first four years of life.

This morbid chain does not end there. The pregnant mother, with small bone size from her own early malnutrition, with poor nutrition and infectious diseases during

[*] January, 1969 testimony of Dr. Charles Upton Lowe to the Senate Select Committee on Nutrition and Human Needs.

pregnancy, is more likely to deliver a premature infant. This child, if it lives, will have greatly increased risks of brain damage, slow development, and other problems.

Spin still another cycle with the malnourished child who is much more susceptible to infection; once infected, he has a more difficult time recovering because of continued poor nutrition. Children suffering from malnutrition develop gastro-intestinal illnesses, including diarrhea, which contribute to more malnutrition and more diarrhea. Likewise, malnutrition and intestinal worms interact to worsen each condition. A South Carolina study showed black children receiving only 50 percent of needed calories, and worms reducing even this inadequate nutrition. The vicious cycle of poverty can be an enduring one, and the evidence is overwhelming that the chain of poverty is intimately connected with mental retardation.

After describing this "morbid chain," Dr. Charles Upton Lowe, a pediatrician and scientific director of the National Institute of Child Health and Human Welfare, told Congress: "The premature birth rate of the poor is three times that of the well-to-do. As many as 50 percent of prematurely born infants grow to maturity with intellectual capacity significantly below normal. The children of the poor show impaired learning ability three to five times as often as other children."

Dr. Joseph English,* former Assistant Director for Health for the Office of Economic Opportunity, approached the vicious cycle of illness and malnutrition from another direction: "Five percent of the children in the United States are born mentally retarded, yet by the time that age group reaches 12 years of age, 11 percent are retarded,

---

* Now administrator of the Health Services and Mental Health Administration within the Department of Health, Education, and Welfare.

which indicates that we *produce* almost as much mental retardation as is born. And when you consider the fact that 75 percent of the mental retardation in this country comes from poor urban and rural areas in poverty and when you consider the role malnutrition can play, then I think you can see how serious this problem is."

Yet many Americans remain skeptical or disbelieving because they do not know that the most devastating effects of malnutrition are unseen, the phenomenon of "hidden hunger." Even though the malnourished person may look normal, his body tissues may be so lacking in essential nutrients that physical output is reduced, resistance to desease is lowered, and body changes occur, affecting both physical growth and mental development. In addition, scientists now conclude that serious protein deficiency can produce physical and mental stunting even though a baby is fed adequate calories. Because most of the very poor in America tend to subsist, by habit and by necessity, on a diet made up largely of starchy foods, low in essential nutrients, the effects of hidden hunger often produce malnourished fat people. In 1967, when Mississippi's Governor Paul Johnson was asked about hunger among the black poor in his state, he scoffed, "All the Negroes I've seen around here are so fat they shine!"

With this callous comment, the former governor may have been pointing unwittingly to one of the signs of a seriously malnourished population.

Scientists who appeared before Congress stressed just that point: The malnourished poor may not *appear* hungry or starved, but their malnutrition may have produced changes in biochemical metabolism of body cells, thereby producing limitations in growth and development. The National Nutrition Survey has found children of poverty lagging six months to 2½ years behind their peers in physical development. And the survey reported that more than a third of all poor children suffer from energy-sapping anemia and shortages of Vitamins A and C.

"The ill-fed among seven million poor American children constitute a danger to the nation, for they may never function in the labor market," Dr. Charles Upton Lowe * told the dozen members of the Senate Select Committee on Nutrition and Human Needs, thus raising another question to the conscience of America: If the American poor are being physically and mentally stunted and weakened by malnutrition, has the War on Poverty, by ignoring a basic problem, wasted the billions it has spent on education and job training? Is it possible, for instance, that even Project Head Start—the popular program for three-to-five year-old children—may be too late?

When President Nixon met with his Urban Affairs Council on March 17, 1969, the conversation centered on this cost. The President asked whether inadequate food really could cause mental retardation, and his staff debated that issue for many weeks. He asked about the cost of a food aid program and his Budget Bureau actually came up with a cost benefit ratio, telling him it would cost only $457 annually to feed a poor child properly, while it would cost the government $1,516 a year per person in welfare, hospitalization, and other expenses to care for the child's later ailments if he went unfed.

Still another question concerns man's social behavior. How does a state of hunger or malnutrition shape a child's —or a man's—attitude toward his world? Talk long enough

---

* Lowe, a top government scientist, in the early 1960's began urging the medical profession to pay more attention to the problems of malnutrition among children. The 47-year-old pediatrician heads the Committee on Nutrition of the American Academy of Pediatrics.

to the "other American" child; ask him what he ate for breakfast; ask him what he did during luchtime at school when the other children bought food, as has Dr. Robert Coles, the gentle Harvard psychiatrist whose great empathy has won the confidence of the poor. He describes what hunger means to children when they are sick most of the time and are regularly hungry:

"They become tired, petulant, suspicious, and finally apathetic. . . . They ask themselves and others what they have done to be kept from the food they want, or what they have done to deserve the pain they seem to feel. . . . the aches and sores of the body become for the child of four or five . . . a reflection of his own worth, and a judgment upon him and his family by the outside world, which he not only feels but judges himself.

"When the rest of us miss a meal or two or experience a stomach ache or injury we are moved to do something about it and succeed in evading the irritability and anger we quite naturally feel. In my experience with families in the Delta, their kind of life can produce a chronic state of mind, a form of withdrawn, sullen behavior."

Dr. Coles' studies took place over a period of eight years in the primitive, rural South. Yet, he describes how the attitudes of the rural poor continue after they migrate north:

"They have more food, more welfare money, and in the public hospitals of the northern city, certain medical services. But one sees how persistently sickness and hunger in children live on into adults who doubt any offer, mistrust any goodness and regard any favorable turn of events as temporary and ultimately unreliable. I fear we have among us now in this country hundreds of thousands of people who have literally grown up to be, and learned

40

to be tired, fearful, anxious, and suspicious and—in a basic and tragic sense—simply unbelieving."

Place the American with these attitudes in a northern city ghetto, where social and racial revolutions burn fiercely, and it will not take long for him to be disillusioned and disabused of his few expectations. As the majority of Americans become wealthier, the poor have become more desperately poor. A great gulf is widening between the poor and the rest of us.

The cost of hunger has been so obscured that many complacent citizens assume that malnutrition is a problem of ignorance, or that hunger exists because of lazy poor people who do not want to work. But the fact is that poor people actually make *better* nutritional use of their money than do the well-to-do (see Chapter VI), and most of the able-bodied poor do work. The ranks of the poor in 1968 included 8.2 million persons in families in which the family head worked full-time, 6.5 million in families with a part-time working family head, 7.6 million in families in which the family leader was elderly or disabled, and only 3.7 million (including 2 million children) in families in which an able-bodied family head was unemployed.

Some cautious scientists and government officials warn that the causal effects of malnutrition cannot be measured, and that judgment must be withheld because hunger is only one factor in the complicated syndrome of poverty. Ill health related to malnutrition may be equally related to unheated housing, lack of sanitation, lack of medical care, of clothing, and the like. The factors involved in the syndrome of poverty are difficult to separate, but failure to reach perfect scientific truths is no excuse for not feeding the hungry. If poverty warriors have learned anything in the 1960s, it is that the culture of poverty is

*41*

indeed complex, and that malnutrition was long over-looked as a factor. If hunger is, in fact, a new metaphor for looking at the problems of abject poverty, it is the most basic one.

"The cost of hunger is too high for continued argument about whether ignorance or poverty is responsible for malnutrition, and too high for delaying action until all the factors can be analyzed in the culture of poverty," stresses Dr. Lowe. "The morbid chain must be broken by assuring that all infants, young children, and pregnant mothers get adequate nutrition."

It is rapidly becoming apparent that one of the costs of hunger in America is the judgment that it leads some men to make about basic American institutions. This judgment is made by Charley Edwards, an elderly Negro who worked for many years on Senator James O. Eastland's Mississippi plantation, and who has had a son in Vietnam:

"He doesn't mind fighting for his country 'cause he was born here and he's been here all his life. He don't mind fighting for it. He don't mind dying for it.

"But to think, if he don't die in Viet Nam, and then comes back here where he lives, he won't feel good over it.

"I think he ought to have some of what he needs. I'd think if I went and took all that punishment, you know, and then came back home and couldn't have a decent bed to lay down in and not a decent job, I don't think I'd feel like this was my country, no space for my part or for me. I'd feel like it was for the other fellow, instead of me."

The basic ethical and moral issue at hand involves the fundamental right of every American to develop to his fullest the physical and mental growth potential within his genetic capacity. "When the authors of the Declaration of Independence wrote that men have the right to life, liberty, and the pursuit of happiness, they probably meant the right not to have a life taken away by execution or incarceration," a former Peace Corps doctor told an American medical convention. "Today, the right to life —for the poor—has a different meaning. It means the right not to have life whittled away by the kinds of illnesses which are the products of poverty."

An indictment of American society was made by hundreds of persons who came to Washington for the Poor People's Campaign in 1968, who shouted "that's right" as the Reverend Ralph David Abernathy told the Secretary of Agriculture, after a year of inaction on food aid to the poor: "That hunger exists is a national disgrace. That so little has been done in the past year to alleviate the known conditions is shocking. It is inequitable to pay large farmers huge amounts of federal funds to grow nothing while poor persons have insufficient amounts to eat."

As the real conditions of American poverty finally were spotlighted, Abernathy and many others began to question the spending priorities in a nation which could find $3 billion to pay farmers not to grow food and yet manage to spend less than one-fifth of that amount to help the hungry poor.

CHAPTER IV

# Let Them Eat Politics
# Origins of the Federal Food Programs

WHEN SENATORS KENNEDY AND CLARK WENT to the Agriculture Department to seek emergency aid for Mississippi, they thought federal food programs were designed to feed poor people—and they came to report that the programs were not working.

What the two senators learned was that those programs were created to help the American farmer boost his prices and get rid of his surplus crops. The hungry poor merely formed one avenue of disposal.

By 1967, less than a million farmers grew most of the nation's food and reaped most of the benefits from federal price support programs. And of these successful commercial farmers, the wealthiest 25 percent received 75 percent of the subsidy payments. The payments might help the small farmer a bit, but only to ease his path as he joined the endless migration off the farm.

Each of the four major food programs managed by the Department of Agriculture was shaped to help the commercial farmer, and all were administered to suit the political conservatism and regional biases of the southern congressmen who controlled the Department's pursestrings and its legislation.

The *Commodity Distribution Program* helps support farm prices by purchasing surplus crops, which are then delivered to the poor through county welfare agencies. The *Food Stamp Program* allows the poor to purchase stamps redeemable for food at grocery stores. The *National School Lunch Program* gives the states money and commodities for nutritious lunches for school children, including free or reduced-priced lunches for poor children. The *Special Milk Program* subsidizes the cost of an extra half pint of milk sold to children at reduced prices.

The first fact Kennedy and Clark learned was that most of the poorest Americans received the benefits from none of these programs. Fewer than 1 of 6 poor Americans benefited at all from the commodity or food stamp programs. Only two million of seven million poor children received the free or reduced-price school lunches to which they were legally entitled. In fact, little of the school lunch and school milk money was spent on poor children.

Next, the senators discovered that all the programs operated inadequately. The surplus commodities—such as flour, cornmeal, and peanut butter—lacked enough calories, vitamins, and minerals for a minimum diet. The food stamps were too costly for most of the poor; for those who could save enough money to participate, the stamps did not provide enough food to meet Department of Agriculture minimum diet requirements.

Because the programs existed at the option of local officials, many counties and school districts denied their poor any food aid. State and local officials also determine eligibility for program benefits, and there is no appeal from even their most arbitrary decisions. When Edgar Cahn, as attorney for the Citizens' Advocate Center, challenged the food stamp law in court, he pointed out that the stamp law and its regulations provided a grocer with a means of appeal if he were excluded from the program, but—incredibly—it gave no means of appeal to the excluded poor. In drafting the program, Department of Agriculture officials had talked to many representatives of the nation's vast agriculture and food handling business, but by their own admission, never consulted with the people the food stamp program was supposed to help—the hungry poor. More than one-half the states deny food aid to many persons with less income than the poverty guideline (in 1967 it was $3,335 for a family of four). This "local option" encourages such eccentric rules as the one in an Indiana township which denies commodity aid to families with dogs in the household. Eligibility requirements for a family of four vary from a maximum of $1,920 income in So. Carolina to a maximum of $4,200 in New York.

Agriculture Department officials had ample evidence of these and other inadequacies in the government's food aid programs long before Senators Clark and Kennedy raised their voices in protest. USDA studies in 1961 and 1962 showed that Blackfeet Indians in Montana, who depended upon the commodity distribution program for survival, were suffering from inadequate nutrition. In 1963, a pilot food stamp study in Cleveland showed that eight of every 10 persons participating had diets rated very poor to poor—"at best, emergency" diets, said one doctor. And, in 1964, a government-wide task force found that the dried skim milk provided in the commodity program did not give infants and expectant mothers the Vitamins A and D they need; task force health experts urged a special commodity package to help them. Five years late, in 1969, such a program finally was started.

Although Agriculture Secretary Orville Freeman was sympathetic to the senators' pleas that he make emergency reforms in the food aid programs, he knew that special welfare aid for the poor—particularly the black poor of the Deep South—would be strongly and bitterly resisted by the agriculture committees of the Congress. These committees and the agriculture appropriations subcommittees are dominated by southern segregationists and midwestern arch-conservatives dedicated to protecting commercial agriculture and opposed to social welfare legislation. Neither the committees nor their chairmen (Senators Allen Ellender of Louisiana and Spessard Holland of Florida; Representatives W. R. Poage of Texas and Jamie Whitten of Mississippi) represent a majority view in Congress, but they reign like feudal barons over the farm policy of the richest agricultural nation in history.

The views of these committees and their power over the department were hardly a darkly held secret, but few urban senators or Washington reporters ever bothered to learn much about the situation or about the food programs. Agriculture represented the mind-boggling "farm problem" to most of Washington's officialdom; liberals avoided it like the plague. For years, congressional food program hearings could have been held in a telephone booth, attended mainly by Department of Agriculture officials and food industry lobbyists. Farm lobbyists busied themselves protecting their particular crop or product and this concern more than once manifested it-

47

self in opposition to programs which might help the hungry poor. The hearings seldom even made a pretense of discussing the general public interest. Few advocates for the poor, or of the public purse, heard the lobbyist for the milk producers and Senator Allen Ellender agree in a 1966 hearing of his committtee that the Special Milk Program should not give first priority to poor children. "The Special Milk Program was for the producer, rather than a program to assist children," stated Agriculture Committee Chairman Ellender.

Liberal members of Congress, by threatening to kill some farm bill favored by conservatives, won the Johnson Administration request for food stamps. The original food stamp bill went through Congress tied to a wheat-cotton bill in 1964, and for the next three years expansions of the program were linked in political trades to legislation supporting southern cotton, peanuts, sugar cane, or tobacco crops. The final bills and their administrative rules were determined by the agriculture committees, and the liberal supporters seldom read the small print. Representative Leonor Sullivan (D., Mo.), the "mother of the food stamp plan," repeatedly ignored its administrative monstrosities, but Mrs. Sullivan had her hands full arranging voting trades to "buy" any food stamp program at all.

Robert Kennedy and Joseph Clark had seen the hunger problem in Mississippi, thought it a simple one, and were amazed that the government seemed unwilling to respond to it. When Orville Freeman delayed and threw up complicated explanations of the limitations on his power to act, Robert Kennedy was incredulous. "I don't know, Orville," he said, describing the sick children. "I'd just get some food down there."

Clark's liberal-dominated Senate Poverty Subcommittee * wrote President Johnson on April 17, 1967, asking for a national program of free food stamps for the neediest, cheaper stamps for the poor, and an investigation of careless or arrogant administration of food programs by local officials. The Senators did not realize it, but their proposal challenged the entire pattern of federal food aid programs which had grown out of Franklin D. Roosevelt's New Deal.

Until the Roaring Twenties collapsed into a depression, few Americans considered it the government's responsibility to help either farmers or poor citizens. When Democratic leader William MacAdoo suggested in 1931 that surplus wheat be distributed to the unemployed, President Hoover flatly disapproved. "I am confident," Hoover said, " that the hungry and unemployed will be cared for by our sense of voluntary organization and community service."

But the economic situation grew darker. Resistance to federal food aid lowered as thousands of farmers, ruined by depression prices, shot hogs, burned grain, and overturned milk trucks, while city dwellers walked the streets penniless and hungry. Finally in 1934, President Roosevelt authorized the Federal Employment Relief Agency to distribute surplus food to the destitute millions on relief. In 1936, another arm was added to the program when Section 32 of Public Law 320 gave the Agriculture Department 30 percent of all customs receipts. The funds were to be used to boost farm prices either by subsidizing exports or by buying overproduced, perishable vegetables and fruit.

* Members of the subcommittee were: Clark, Kennedy, Javits, Murphy, Jennings Randolph (D.,W.Va.), Claiborne Pell (D., R.I.), Edward Kennedy (D.,Mass.), and Winston Prouty (R., Vt.).

49

By 1939, 13 million Americans were eating surplus food.

From 1939 to 1943, the Agriculture Department operated a complicated food stamp program for the farmer by feeding his surplus products into the mouths of the poor via the marketplace. When World War II brought prosperity to the farmer and jobs to the unemployed, federal food aid stopped, but as soon as the war ended, farmers were again wrestling with price-depressing surpluses. Mechanization, new seeds and fertilizer, good weather, and added manpower produced bumper crops. The agriculture committees stepped in to help the farmer with the 1946 National School Lunch Act, with a Food for Peace Program for surplus food aid overseas, and with an additional authorization in 1949 to purchase overproduced commodities for distribution to the poor or to schools.

The Commodity Distribution Program expanded rapidly after the Department of Agriculture agreed in 1953 to pay shipping costs to the states. By 1959, when the program reached 1,300 counties, it provided a family of four with 20 pounds of flour, ten pounds of corn meal, nine pounds of nonfortified dried milk, two pounds of rice, and occassionally, four pounds of butter and ten pounds of cheese per month. Where states and counties exercised their local option not to take certain items, the variety of foodstuffs might be less. There was no meat, limited protein and calories, and no vitamin C. Even the most ingenious housewife could not maintain adequate nutrition in her family on this fare.

By 1959 the nation was floundering in an economic recession, and out-of-work coalminers in Appalachia appealed for more food aid. As he sought to help his Kentucky constituents, Republican Senator John Sherman Cooper realized that Agriculture Secretary Ezra Taft Benson, in administering the commodity program, gave *last* priority to the needs of hungry poor Americans. Finding that huge amounts of cooking oils were stored in government tanks, Cooper asked why they could not be distributed to the hungry poor in his state. They were being held for overseas sales, Benson told him, as he spelled out government policy: First priority was overseas sale for dollars; second priority was Food for Peace sale with payment in soft foreign currency for American use overseas. Benson was carrying out the mandates of the congressional committees, as was his undersecretary, who met another request to help unemployed workers by saying, "We are most sympathetic to the plight of needy persons. We must, however, not lose sight of the fact that the primary responsibility of the Department is to carry out the farm programs that benefit farmers."

Indeed, there is no mention of the needs of hungry Americans in the official Department of Agriculture statement of policy on disposal of commodities. The needs of the poor obviously did not matter to Agriculture Department officials, who negotiated agreements with each of the states on how the programs would be run. These quiet contracts served the interests of everyone but the poor. Most farm states provided commodities only in the nonfarming season, and some, such as Arizona, specifically ruled that a family with a potential farm worker in it could not be eligible as long as farm work was available in Arizona or any of the surrounding states. The eligibility requirements varied widely. In Louisiana, for example, a family of four could obtain commodities only if its income were $165 per month or less. The Agriculture Department exercised little supervision over local politicians, who gave or withheld food at their whim. If the poor could surmount all these obstacles, their only problem would be transportation to pick up the commodities, and inspiration to figure out how to prepare a menu confined to three staple food grains and some occasional cheese.

After President Kennedy doubled the number of foods in the commodity program, and even after the commodity list was increased to 15 items during the Johnson administration, the program remained nutritionally inadequate. Even if the counties took all the items, which most did not (including Chairman Bob Poage's and Lyndon Johnson's Texas), the commodity diet still lacked enough calories and important vitamins. Rodney Leonard, Department of Agriculture administrator of food programs in 1967-1968, admitted he had been at his job almost a year before learning that most counties did not take all offered commodities. The Agriculture Department placed a low priority on disseminating information on food aid services.

In his first month in office, President Kennedy ordered that a pilot food stamp program (authorized in 1959 but never used by President Eisenhower) be set into operation. Congress legislated a food stamp program in 1964 and the money authorization climbed from $75 million in 1965 to $100 million in 1966, $200 million for 1967 and 1968, and $225 million for 1969.

In theory, the food stamp plan *sounded* simple and workable, and should have been an enormous improvement over commodity distribution. The eligible poor pay the government the amount of money that they normally spend for food every month. In exchange, they receive stamps of this value plus bonus stamps that permit them to buy extra food. Grocery stores accept the stamps as money and redeem them from the government.

In practice, though, the food stamp plan amounted to

virtual extortion from the poor; it was no accident that the stamp payment formula produced the outcries "We can't afford the stamps" and "The stamps run out after two weeks." Following their congressional leaders' twin desires of helping the farmers but not providing welfare to the poor, Agriculture Department bureaucrats had designed a food stamp program so conservative that reformers called the plan "Scrooge stamps."

There was no doubt as to the motives of congressmen who run the Agriculture Department. Testifying on the proposed food stamp law before the Senate Agriculture Committee in 1964, one Agriculture Department official boldly suggested that it would not help those with little or no income, but Committee Chairman Ellender indignantly dismissed this complaint against the bill. "I know that in my state we had a number of fishermen who were unable to catch fish," retorted Ellender. "Do you expect the government, because they cannot catch fish, to feed them until the fish are there?" In other words, this food stamp program is not to be considered a program just simply to feed people because they cannot get work. This is not what it is supposed to be."

According to Ellender's anti-welfare principles, the program was supposed to increase food consumption by charging so much for the stamps that any person participating actually had to sacrifice other necessities to gain more food for his family.

The Food Stamp Program had been advocated by Agriculture Department economists with the rationale that it would provide more monetary benefits to the farmer than did the commodity programs. Economists reasoned that the poor would spend their meager dollars for cheap grains such as wheat, corn, and rice, even though they did not get these products free. The way to insure use of other farm commodities, therefore, would be to encourage the poor to buy more food.

The amount of money a family must pay is based on the monthly income and the number of persons in a family. For example, according to the rigid calculations of the Department of Agriculture, a mother with three dependent children, whose sole income was a $70 monthly welfare check (a common figure in the South), paid $34 to receive $64 worth of grocery-buying food stamps in 1967, leaving her $36 for rent, utilities, clothing, medicine, and other expenses. She was forced to pay almost 50 percent of her income for stamps—an inordinate amount, considering that the average American spends only 17 percent of income for food. Furthermore, even the Department of Agriculture admits that $64 worth of food would not be enough. The Department contends that a family of four needs at least $100 worth of groceries a month to maintain a minimum diet, while it considers $120 a more realistic figure. Supplying this family with only 64/100 of a survival diet led to bitter charges of "government-mandated" hunger.

Another hardship was that stamps had to be purchased in a lump sum on a monthly or bi-monthly basis. Anyone with a realistic conception of extreme poverty knows that most families with $70, $100, or even $200 monthly incomes must spend money as they get it. As the pressure builds to cover necessities such as rent, doctor bills, or a pair of shoes so a child can go to school, the budget for food often is whatever money is left. If the family with limited but regular income has trouble saving for the lump sum payments, the family with irregular income finds it impossible. In order to participate in the program, families were required to pay an amount equivalent to their "normal expenditure for food," but in reality the very poor have *no* "normal" expenditure. (Small wonder Mississippi Negroes shouted that the switch from inadequate but free surplus commodities to inaccessibly priced food stamps was a move to drive them out of the state.)

As counties throughout the nation changed from free commodities to food stamps, participation in the government programs fell off by 40 percent; more than one million persons, including 100,000 in Mississippi, were forced to drop out of the food aid program. The average participation rate of poor persons in areas where food stamps are available is only 16 percent. Aside from the stigma of poverty that keeps proud men away from food stamps, this low participation rate reflects the costliness and limited benefits of the program, as well as the lack of information about the program, the inaccessibility of food stamp centers, and the blatant discrimination in running the program.

The formula seemed to work on the assumption that the poorer a family was, the less food it was supposed to need to eat. Confounded by this discriminatory difference, Representative Albert Quie of Minnesota asked Agriculture Secretary Freeman: "Are his [the poorest person's] nutritional needs different?"

Replied Freeman: "His nutritional needs, I expect, are probably the same. His food habits, however, are sharply different. . . . The strong likelihood is . . . [that] a significant number of these stamps would be bootlegged." The planners hoped to insure against "bootlegging" (trading stamps for cash, soap, or other items) by allowing the poorest man so few stamps that he would need them all to feed his family.

Secretary Freeman was eager to assure the Agriculture Department's congressional bosses that the farmer's benefits would not be risked in favor of more federal help for the very poorest, who might just divert the stamps to other needs. In this argument, he accepted the convenient myth that the poor somehow are too ignorant to want the right food for themselves and their children, and, therefore, cannot be trusted to use a liberalized program—a myth cherished by Chairmen Ellender, Poage, Holland, and Whitten.

At every turn, Freeman appeared to mold and defend the Department's food programs in terms calculated to soothe his congressional overseers. When asked to liberalize the Food Stamp Program so that the very poorest would be able to afford the stamps, he argued (in 1967 congressional testimony) that free or cheaper stamps would mean that the states would contribute less to relief. "They [the states] cannot use the food stamp program as a backdoor method of shifting that responsibility [i.e., welfare] to the Department of Agriculture," he said.

Vigorously arguing that the Food Stamp Program must remain a "food" program and not contain any vestige of a "welfare" break for the poor, former Minnesota Governor Freeman began to sound more and more like conservative Louisianan Allen Ellender.

When he testified before the agriculture committees, Freeman stressed that the farmer got $2.01 per week from a Food Stamp Program participant versus only $1.75 per person in the Commodity Distribution Program. Similar statistics were not prepared to compare the diet possible with food stamps to the nutritional needs of human beings.

At a time when hundreds of counties with hungry poor competed to get in the Food Stamp Program, Freeman's congressional relations men helped pick the priority counties on the basis of congressional politics. Such politicking is not unusual in Washington; it is merely shocking when applied to human survival.

A few days before he left office, Freeman finally admitted to Congress that his department had charged too much for food stamps and given out too few bonus stamps. But he attributed the stinginess of the food stamp formula to a tight budget.

If Freeman felt that he had to knuckle under to the southern conservatives and segregationists, he at least had good cause for concern. The Food Stamp Program had always been approved by only the narrowest margin and only then in a deal with the southerners. Perhaps he reflected that only a highly conservative program could escape criticism and survive. At one point in 1967 he asked Joseph Clark to stop criticizing the programs until his appropriations had safely passed Congress.

With some bitterness, Freeman noted that the hunger crusaders were nowhere to be found when he had attempted to reform food programs in earlier years. The Secretary had just cause for complaint, although he never tried to rally public support for controversial food reforms opposed by the committees that govern his department.

Because the White House, the public, and most of the Congress were not yet informed or aroused, Orville Freeman's few pre-1967 attempts to improve the food programs rarely got the approval of a congressional committee. Such was the case in 1966 when the Johnson Administration, in its proposed Child Nutrition Act, sought to give priority treatment to poor children in benefits from the Special Milk Program. No one raised a word of protest as Chairman Ellender and Patrick Healy, a lobbyist for the National Milk Producers Association, cynically discussed the real purpose of the milk program—a purpose they did not want endangered politically by any priorities for the poor. The purpose was to help the milk industry, not to help children.

As with the Special Milk Program, the National School Lunch Program also was shaped to meet the needs of commercial agriculture and the conservative philosophies of the agriculture committees. Steered through Congress in 1946 by Senators Ellender and Richard Russell, the law was supposed to supply every American child, rich or poor, with a hot, nutritious meal at school. The law states that the poor are to receive their lunches free, or at reduced prices. However, neither the rich nor the poor are served adequately by the program. After studying the school lunch program in 1969, a panel of the nation's outstanding nutritionists expressed shock at the high fat and low protein content of many school meals. (The panel found ¾ of the meals lacked adequate calories, ⅝ lacked sufficient iron and magnesium, and ⅛ were short on essential vitamins. It recommended improving the school lunch diet by fortification and enrichment of foods, and by employing the services of skilled outside catering firms.)

In 1967 at least four million poor children from families with less than $2,000 annual income were denied the free or reduced-price lunches theoretically guaranteed them by law. In fact, only 19 million out of 50 million American school children participated at all in the 1967 program. The law requires that the individual states must spend $3 for every $1 of federal aid, but fewer than a dozen states meet this requirement. Most school districts use the money paid by students—usually 25 to 40 cents daily—to account for the state's share of spending in the program.

Poor children suffer especially because several thousand American schools, with 9 million students, have no facilities for providing school lunches. More often than not, these are older ghetto schools in America's largest central cities or poor rural schools—the schools containing the most poor children. Boston, which likes to think of itself as "the cradle of learning," had perhaps the worst program, rivaled only by Philadelphia and Detroit in the failure to provide lunches to most poor children. Many school boards were philosophically opposed to providing school children with free lunches. Others never could fit food programs into perpetually inadequate budgets. Teachers often opposed the program because they would be required to serve "lunch duty." In most urban neighborhoods, schools have no kitchens because children traditionally walked home for lunch. Today, many of these neighborhoods are ghettoes where a high percentage of mothers are away from home during the day.

The problem of older, city schools without food facilities could have been eased years ago by employing outside food catering firms who were eager for the business. For 22 years, however, this idea was blocked by a powerful but little-known lobby of school lunch administrators, the American Food Service Association.

The school lunch administrators, who feared private caterers would eliminate their jobs, also lobbied against earmarking federal funds to feed free meals to poor children. The administrators contended they would take care of poor children out of general federal school lunch aid, yet they had provided free lunches to only two million out of about six or seven million poor children.

When Congress debated extending the lunch program to provide meals for poor pre-schoolers in such places as day care centers, Ellender and his colleagues blasted the proposal because it would "make the school lunch program into a welfare program. . . . This could lead to the demand for greater federal funds," he complained.

As it now operates, the school lunch program is hardly a welfare program. Poor children from one end of the nation to the other are subjected to humiliating discrimination in applying for and receiving free lunches. In some schools, children are required to stand aside and let paying students go first. In others, children are humiliated by having to use lunch tickets of a different color from those used by fellow students, or, contrary to law, by being required to work for their meals. Methods of determining which children receive free or reduced-price meals vary widely from city to city and even within the same school district. Most schools are so short of funds that poor children must take turns having a free meal. In other schools, the hungry poor must sit in the cafeteria and watch other children eat. Because of a shortage of both federal and local lunch funds, many schools use funds from the Elementary and Secondary Education Act to pay for free lunches—money which really should be used to improve educational opportunity for poor children.

As outside criticism of Department of Agriculture programs mounted, Orville Freeman became adamant in defending his department's policies. Yet if any group kept Orville Freeman aware of faulty government food aid programs, it was his own advisory committee on civil rights. Freeman appointed the committee in 1965, after President Johnson and the U. S. Commission on Civil Rights had chided the Agriculture Department for gross discrimination in both its programs and its hiring practices. From the beginning, the committee—led by the late Ralph McGill, editor of the Atlanta *Constitution,* and poverty worker Clay Cochran—petitioned Freeman to liberalize the food stamp and commodity programs, to put in federal food aid where local officials refused to help the hungry, and to free the school lunch program from segregationist politics.

It took only a few trips through the South for the committee to see how that region's politicians succeeded in bending food programs to serve the needs of the South's segregationist politics and cotton economics. School lunch funds were used blatantly to maintain segregation. In an effort to discourage poor Negro parents from sending their children to white schools, no free meals would be provided at those schools—but free lunches suddenly sprang up in the all-Negro schools.

The civil rights advisory committee was convinced that the switchover from commodities to food stamps was part of a new effort to drive the Negro out of the South. Ironically, conditions for white planters and Negro farm workers were not much different in the 1960s than they had been in 1934, when Congress, prodded by the southern planters on the agriculture committees, passed farm laws sharply cutting back cotton production. As was the case again in 1965, these laws were designed without any regard to their effect on human beings. Thrown out of what little work they had, Negroes either went north or went hungry. But in 1965, such a policy was far less justified than it had been in 1934, when several million farmers still shared in the crop retirement payments. By 1965 most of the small farmers were gone, and the payments went to huge plantation owners. During the 32 years since the New Deal first promised help to the farmer, the programs had only compounded the problems of the farm laborer. The President's Commission on Rural Poverty criticized the department for not even considering the effect on farm labor in drafting the 1965 program cutting back cotton production. By considering only crops and not poor people, the commission said, the Department of Agriculture was contributing to hunger and poverty.

Since Freeman refused to correct inequities and discrimination in food aid, his civil rights advisory committee asked that he at least supply them with the facts, so they could take the case to the public. In response, Freeman placed his advisory committee under the care of an aide, Kenneth Birkhead, whose explicit job was to smooth over (and, hopefully, silence) race and poverty issues that might irritate committee chairmen Whitten, Holland, Poage, and Ellender.

Frustrated at its own inability to force the Agriculture Department to collect pertinent data which would show the effectiveness of its food programs, the U. S. Commission on Civil Rights finally wrote to Freeman's civil rights aide, William Seabron: "We note that the Consumer and Marketing Service has developed data collection systems which can inform it of the number of pounds of selected types of cigar wrapper tobacco products each year, as well as the number of pounds of goat meat condemned after reinspection for being tainted, sour, or putrid. We ask only that the same amount of imagination that can develop a system to collect data such as this be applied to the critical area of equal opportunity and program participation in food programs."

The total administration of food and welfare programs from the national to the local level seemed designed—consciously or unconsciously—to limit participation. Residency requirements, complicated certification processes, limitation of funds, and inaccessibility of officials all combined to keep people out of programs rather than to help them.

America's crying needs have a habit of losing their identity in Washington. In a process where power, not need, usually dictates, the government's leaders cite bloodless statistics to rationalize the token appropriations they offer to be divided among millons of suffering Americans. In the case of the Agriculture Department food programs, the bureaucrats either feared that alerting the public would antagonize the conservative committees, or else they just didn't want to be bothered. After all, the Department of Agriculture had its hands full with the problems of millions of farmers who also needed aid.

Although the programs were advertised as the salvation of the family farmer, four-fifths of the benefits went to the wealthiest farmers, and more than one million of the smallest farmers received scarcely any help at all. As a vivid example, the largest 264 commercial farms in 1968 received $52 million in payments, as did the 540,000 smallest farms. This meant an average government payment of $197,000 to the wealthy farmers, an average of $96 for the half-million small farmers. The programs were designed to cope with the big farmer's acreage problems, and the poorest farmers suffered almost as much as did the exploited farm laborer.

In uncovering the thinking that had tailored all the government's food programs, Senators Kennedy and Clark discovered, as others had before, that these programs were designed and controlled by people who never even considered how their clients were affected. Most of all, the Department of Agriculture bureaucrats never considered the rights of the poor, their personal desires, or their possible knowledge about the problems of poverty. The School Lunch Program, for example, received no congressional examination for 15 years except from appropriations subcommittees whose most influential members flatly opposed more food aid for poor school children. Agriculture Department food administrator Rodney Leonard admitted (after he left office) that department bureaucrats never felt challenged to think about the programs in terms of service to children.

When Senators Kennedy and Clark pressured Orville Freeman to consider the desperate needs of the poor, the Secretary of Agriculture found himself caught between two conflicting forces—the conservative, controlling committees of Congress, and the influential voices of a new breed of liberals who believed a War on Poverty meant far more than the traditional and inadequate dole. It should mean, they felt, full participation in society—as equal human beings who have the same rights of dignity, self-determination, and political participation.

How the Secretary of Agriculture handled this power struggle would be the story of Round One in the new politics of hunger.

# CHAPTER V

# The Politics of Hunger—Round One

FOR ORVILLE FREEMAN, THE SQUEEZE WAS ON.
From the morning of April 13, 1967, when Robert F. Kennedy and Joseph Clark walked into his office, the Secretary of Agriculture took a constant shelling from liberal advocates demanding immediate action for the hungry poor people in Mississippi. Pressure from the other side also was building. His Appropriations Subcommittee Chairman Jamie Whitten and Senate Agriculture member James O. Eastland both were furious at the exposure of conditions in their state by a coalition of northern liberals and southern blacks. The southerners, who dominated Freeman's congressional committees both in influence and in numbers, regarded increasing food aid for Negroes as dangerous. They warned the Secretary not to tamper with the social and economic structure of the South.

With one eye on the national attention commanded by the junior Senator from New York, veteran politician Orville Freeman carefully balanced the political toll from an all-out Kennedy attack on the Department of Agriculture against the future of the Department's legislative programs at the hands of wrathful congressional committees. Until Freeman received definite direction from the White House, all decisions regarding food programs were his. And the President, preoccupied with Vietnam, gave low priority to problems at Agriculture.

Immediately after the Kennedy-Clark visit to his office, Freeman dispatched two aides to the Mississippi Delta to give him a personal report on the situation. Peter Edelman,* Kennedy's 29-year-old legislative assistant, accompanied them, retracing the steps of the senators' earlier trip.

As he led Agriculture Department officials Howard Davis and William Seabron through the Delta, Edelman was determined to disprove the department's claim that all families could scrape up the minimum cost ($2 a month per person) of food stamps. After a tiring day of visiting shacks, career bureaucrat Davis commented, "We've seen enough; let's head back to Washington."

"But you haven't seen everything," protested Edelman. "There's much more."

The officials replied that they had seen enough to make an accurate judgment on hunger conditions, and Edelman demanded to know whether they were now satisfied that

* Three years earlier the Minneapolis-born Edelman had been heading toward a Wall Street law practice after having attended Harvard Law School and served as a Supreme Court law clerk. He detoured for a few months to work in Kennedy's 1964 senatorial campaign, and became involved in the struggle for social reform.

66

many persons had no income with which to purchase food stamps.

"We're satisfied," replied food administrator Davis.

At the same time, Freeman sent a team of nutritionists to Mississippi to weigh the adequacy of food programs. They soon reported that existing programs provided only minimal help to the poor. Those people in the food stamp program, those in the commodity program, and those receiving no government aid all fared badly, with only small variations. *Their diet was uniformly worse than had been that of the average southern family with less than $2,000 annual income in 1955—12 years earlier.*

Armed with this kind of information, members of the Senate Poverty Subcommittee attempted to involve President Lyndon Johnson. On April 27, all nine members of the Subcommittee petitioned the President to declare an emergency. Attempting to insure that the letter actually would reach Johnson's eyes; Subcommittee Counsel William Smith called Presidential Assistant Joseph Califano. The letter should be sent to Sargent Shriver (director of the Office of Economic Opportunity), Califano insisted.

"Send it to the White House anyway," Bob Kennedy snapped, when Smith relayed Califano's instructions. Although the senators tried repeatedly to get personal attention from the President, the White House never replied. The first response from the Johnson Administration came in the form of a bland press release from the Office of Economic Opportunity.

OEO acknowledged problems in Mississippi, but contended more had been done for this state than for other needy areas. "The emergency in Mississippi should not blind us to emergencies elsewhere in America," read the statement, which went on to blame Congress for limiting the War on Poverty. Kennedy's and Clark's pleas for emergency action were ignored. In effect, OEO said Americans can go hungry and the U. S. government cannot respond.

An enraged Robert Kennedy, along with chairman Joe Clark, protested to Shriver, who soon turned up a one-million dollar, four-month emergency loan program so that the poor in 20 counties—including four in Mississippi —could borrow money to buy food stamps. This was merely a symbolic gesture, not even a band-aid over the gaping wound of hunger. Yet it was an admission that the poor could not afford food stamps.

Meanwhile, Kennedy and Clark kept bombarding Secretary Freeman with ways he could use his office to help the hungry poor. There were phone calls, letters, and meetings with the liberals, and at one point Bill Smith almost convinced Freeman of the Secretary's legal powers to help the hungry. Orville Freeman finally acknowledged privately that he had the authority to issue free food stamps and to declare an emergency so commodities could be distributed again in counties where thousands of poor people could not afford food stamps.

The Secretary, however, declined to use these powers until he had checked with Jamie Whitten, the congressman who ruled on his Department's budget.

"No!" thundered the Mississippian, both to free stamps and to having both food stamps and commodity programs in the same counties. The other agriculture committee chairmen (southerners Ellender, Poage, and Hollander) shared Whitten's reluctance. Freeman's total budget for 1968 was under consideration, and he implored Kennedy and Clark not to press him publicly for reforms until the Department's appropriations bill and food stamp extension bill had safely passed the Congress. A belligerent Chairman Poage was holding up an extension of the food program—a mere extension without any of the reforms now being pushed at him by Kennedy and Clark. Freeman seemed to reason that the southerners would just kill the stamp program altogether if they thought he was going to liberalize it. He was playing the old politics, hoping Congresswoman Leonor Sullivan could work up another quiet trade. In the end she did. After showing she could block a peanut bill important to Poage and a handful of other southern congressmen, she was able to secure Poage's support of a two-year food stamp extension. Mrs. Sullivan won renewal of the inadequate program but did not even seek reforms in it.

Finally, in June 1967, nearly two months after the senators called on him for emergency action, Freeman came up with a plan that satisfied no one.

The price of stamps to the poorest families—less than 10 percent of the participants—was reduced from $2 monthly to 50 cents per person; stamps would be half price the first month; poor people would be hired as aides to seek out the hungry to participate; and local welfare authorities would be encouraged to provide food stamp funds for the destitute.

There would be no free stamps, no reduced stamp prices for the bulk of needy families (those with $50 to $150 monthly income), no declaration of an emergency to distribute commodities to those who could not afford food stamps. It was, at best, a conservative compromise.

"Orville was being subjected to pressure by us," Bob Kennedy analyzed later, "but he was much more worried about his own programs, for which he had to answer to Whitten, Eastland, and that crowd. It boiled down to whether we could exert more pressure than the southerners—and we didn't."

Two weeks later, in mid-June, Freeman confirmed that

he was taking his cues from the southern politicians. On a "rural development" trip to Alabama and Mississippi, he carefully avoided the squalor and hopelessness that the two northern senators had seen. The Secretary took a white-guided tour of plantations, staged antiseptic meetings with mostly white audiences, and experienced only one or two unplanned confrontations forced upon him by victims of discrimination. Poverty had initially been on his tour agenda, but calls from Mississippi and Alabama congressmen had changed most of that.

He did visit a few carefully selected shacks, but then refused to stop even for five minutes to greet Negro members of the Southwest Alabama Farmers Cooperative, a federally financed antipoverty project which was guardedly supported by the Department of Agriculture but opposed by every white politician in the state. He announced publicly a federal grant for a new vegetable processing plant in Mississippi that would mainly benefit rich Delta farmers, and met only privately to hear the grievances of Mississippi civil rights leaders about the food stamp program. He whispered to them his modest reforms. Only because they surrounded his bus did he hear a group of Alabama Negroes complain about discrimination in food and other agricultural programs administered by his department. Fifteen minutes later, he told an Alabama reporter that he had heard no complaints about unfair administration of the food programs.

When he returned from Mississippi and Alabama, Freeman clashed with Kennedy, Clark, and Javits on still another issue. The hunger advocates had been pressing him to spend some of Agriculture's Section 32 funds—the department's share of customs receipts—for emergency aid. More than $500 million of these funds had accumulated in the Agriculture Department, which could only carry forward $300 million from one fiscal year to the next. Rather than use any of this money for the poor, however, Freeman returned $200 million to the U. S. Treasury on July 1.

The Poverty Subcommittee was astonished. "How can you return such amounts of money to the Treasury when there are hungry to be fed?" asked Javits.

The Secretary explained that he could only use these Section 32 funds to buy perishable commodities such as beef, pork, citrus fruits, or vegetables when market prices fell below 90 percent of parity (the ratio between what farmers pay for goods and what they receive for their products). His hands were tied, he maintained. (Two years later, former Agriculture Undersecretary John Schnittker would state that virtually all crops could have been bought legally with the funds.)

It was the certain wrath of appropriations chairmen Holland and Whitten, rather than the technicalities of the law, that most concerned Freeman. Both congressional chairmen felt that the Section 32 customs receipts should be used to buy perishables *only* when an oversupply threatened farmers' profits. In fact, the funds are often spent as political pressure dictates, and that is usually to keep big agriculture happy. Such was the case in 1964 and 1965 when the government bought huge quantities of beef with Section 32 funds after cattlemen began pressing for a protective quota on imports. "Surplus foods are what the lawyers say they are," Rodney Leonard, Freeman's administrator for food programs, privately confessed. "We begin buying off commodities from whatever commodity group has enough muscle to get included."

If citrus growers in Senator Holland's Florida produced too many oranges, so that profitable prices were threatened, then children in the school lunch program might drown in orange juice. If the price of orange juice were high, then they would have orange juice only if the local school budget could afford it. (Freeman also was not averse to do a little trading of his own with Section 32 funds. A year later when he sought action on a food aid program, Freeman held out the bait of Section 32 purchase of sugar cane—including some grown in Louisiana—to whet Senator Ellender's appetite for approving a food aid bill.)

Freeman's best defense on returning the Section 32 money to the Treasury was that he merely carried out the Johnson Administration's planned budget. The huge surplus had been anticipated and already was counted as "income" in President Johnson's strict budget. Without orders from the White House and the Budget Bureau, and knowing the congressional attitudes in 1967, Freeman made no effort to bend the budget to meet the emergency.

When the Poverty Subcommittee hearings opened, the senators found Freeman explosively defensive at criticisms of the food programs. The poor had little muscle and the Poverty Subcommittee learned that the Secretary of Agriculture had done all the giving he was going to do.

The hunger hearings on July 11 and 12, 1967, also brought together the Field Foundation doctors, the Surgeon General of the U.S. Public Health Service, and OEO Director Sargent Shriver to testify on the situation in Mississippi.

Debate centered on whether there actually was an emergency. The poignant testimony of the Field Foundation doctors, a month after they had examined the diseased, hungry children in Head Start centers, infuriated Mississippi Senators Eastland and Stennis, who were invited by Clark to sit with the committee.

72

North Carolina physician Raymond Wheeler charged that the white establishment in Mississippi seemed bent on driving Negroes out of the state.

"Gross libel and slander," retorted Stennis.

"Totally untrue," replied Eastland, whose Mississippi state health officials thumbed their noses at "outside agitating doctors" and "quickie experts on Mississippi health."

In reply, Dr. Wheeler looked straight at the Mississippi senators and stated softly:

"I am distressed and concerned that Senators Stennis and Eastland interpret my remarks as libelous to the state of Mississippi. I was born and reared and educated in the South. I love the region.

"Throughout these years my heart has wept for the South as I have watched the southern Negro and the southern white walk their separate ways, distrusting each other, separated by false and ridiculous barriers, doomed to a way of life tragically less than they deserve, when by working together, they could achieve a society finer and more successful than any which exists today in this country.

"Throughout all that dreadful pageant of ignorance and suspicion and mutual distrust, the most distressing figure of all has been the southern political leader who has exploited all our human weaknesses for his own personal and selfish gains, refusing to grant us the dignity and capability of responding to courageous and noble leadership when all of us had nothing to lose but the misery and the desolation which surrounds all our lives.

"The time has come when this must cease, for we are now concerned with little children whose one chance for a healthy, productive, dignified existence is at stake.

"I invite Senators Eastland and Stennis to come with me

into the vast farmlands of the Delta, and I will show them the children of whom we have spoken. I will show them their bright eyes and innocent faces, their shriveled arms and swollen bellies, their sickness and pain, and the misery of their parents.

"Their story must be believed, not only for their sakes, but for the sake of all America."

The huge auditorium in the new Senate Office Building was silent. Then Senator Clark, his voice unsteady, asked, "Senator Eastland, would you care to ask any questions?"

"I have no questions," Senator Eastland replied.

"Senator Stennis?" Clark asked.

"I have no questions," answered Stennis.

On July 21, just 10 days after Dr. Wheeler had left the Mississippi senators temporarily speechless, John Stennis introduced an emergency food and medical bill to the Senate.

The junior Mississippi senator, after expressing grave doubt that anyone really was suffering in his state, said, "What they need is help, not talk and publicity . . . ; they need to be made well, not made the subject of partisan politics or a nationwide television show."

The Stennis bill authorized $10 million for the Agriculture Department and Public Health Service to meet emergency hunger or medical problems.

Frustrated by the three-month battle to get Freeman to act, Kennedy and Clark quickly threw their forces behind the Stennis bill. In a lightning-fast move to seize the legislative opening provided by Stennis, Counsel Bill Smith tracked down committee members all over the country and by day's end every member of the Poverty Subcommittee was listed as a co-sponsor of the Stennis bill. Four days later, Stennis was surprised to learn that

74

the Subcommittee was meeting to act on his legislation. Not expecting such instant response, he begged for a delay because he had not discussed the bill with either Senator Eastland or Mississippi's Governor Paul Johnson, but Clark said "nothing doing" and voted the bill out of committee. Ten days after the bill had been introduced, the Senate approved it, after first increasing its authorization to $25 million the first year and $50 million the second, and adding an authority for a national nutrition survey.

The bill was expected to sail through the House—or so it seemed. Senators Stennis and Clark, working in uneasy tandem, lined up both Mississippi conservatives and northern liberals to support the bill in the House. However, no one had reckoned with the Chairman of the House Agriculture Committee, Bob Poage. A 69-year-old lawyer from Waco, Texas, Poage was considered a populist when he first came to Congress in 1936. In 1967 his populism extended to fervent support of liberal government benefits for farmers in his district. When it came to matters of liberal aid for the poor, Poage became an unreconstructed nineteenth-century conservative who thought both Stennis and the liberals were dallying in a lot of demagogic, welfare politics. He determined to kill the bill in his committee. At a private committee meeting on September 29, the burly committee chairman, whose volcanic temper is well-known in the House, was so rude to the courtly Senator Stennis that he embarrassed his own committee members, particularly fellow southerners.

There was no lobby behind the Stennis bill. The liberals underestimated the potential of the budding hunger issue and had not even introduced legislation. Few northern liberals wanted to work for a bill with Stennis's name on it, and Johnson Administration officials were silent. Almost by default, Robert Choate of the Citizens' Crusade Against Poverty became the bill's sole lobbyist.

And Choate, then a neophyte at congressional lobbying, made a crucial Washington mistake. A public hearing on the bill had been scheduled, but several smooth-talking southern politicians convinced Choate that the bill would zip through the House Agriculture Committee. The committee just wanted to handle it with as little publicity as possible, Choate was told. He agreed to call off his witnesses, leaving Chairman Poage free to cancel the public hearing—which Poage promptly did.

The committee held another private meeting on October 5, at which Poage ranted and raved at Agriculture, HEW, and Bureau of the Budget representatives. "This program is so loosely drawn I can get food from it when my wife is out of town," he yelled. (He did not mention the fact that food aid laws are so tightly drawn that Bell County officials in his own congressional district could deny all food aid to the poor, or the fact that at the same time 68 Bell County farmers were paid $473,000 for not growing crops.)

The Agriculture Department witnesses, intimidated by Poage's outbursts, appeared muddled in their testimony. Food administrator Rodney Leonard gave such weak testimony (he agreed that Poage could get fed by the legislation) that liberal Representative Joseph Resnick stormed from the hearing charging that the Agriculture Department was trying to kill the bill. Leonard and HEW witnesses were afraid to support the legislation enthusiastically without firm instructions from the White House —and there had been no instructions. A majority of the House Agriculture Committee appreciated Poage's performance and crushed the bill by a 22–7 vote. Only

Resnick and Thomas Foley of Washington really fought for it. Congressman Foley, a 39-year-old attorney from Spokane, continued to push the Stennis bill and other food aid reform measures within this solidly conservative committee. The 15 southern Democrats and 15 conservative Republicans, mostly from the Midwest, had demonstrated their common opposition to social reform in a coalition that has a common interest in protecting agriculture and is seldom split by partisan politics. Chairman Poage, a Democrat, and ranking Republican Page Belcher of Oklahoma, the closest of allies, worked together to defeat the Stennis bill.

The coolness toward the Stennis bill by Johnson Administration officials stemmed from a number of reasons. Admission of the need for legislation implied that they were not doing their own jobs well, and the officials felt sensitive to criticism. The White House had not flatly said "no" to the legislation, but the President had not said "yes" either. Knowing how desperately the President wanted to make anti-inflationary budget cuts and how strongly he disliked Robert Kennedy, the officials had two good reasons for being cautious. Lyndon Johnson's volatile personality had been imprinted on enough Cabinet and Subcabinet officers that none ventured to ask what the President might consider an unpleasant question. Lyndon Johnson had quite a temper, and some Cabinet officers preferred to leave decisions hanging rather than risk provoking him. But behind the scenes, the executive branch of a warring Johnson Administration was engaged in significant political maneuvering.

When Senator Clark had adjourned his poverty hearings on July 12, he ordered the Departments of Health, Education, and Welfare and Agriculture, as well as the Office of Economic Opportunity, to report back to the committee within 30 days, detailing the nature of the domestic hunger problem and giving immediate steps to remedy it. Kennedy and Clark had also stimulated OEO Director Sargent Shriver into separate action on the issue, as had Shriver's own staff, who distrusted the farm-oriented officials at Agriculture. Shriver immediately planned a bold response to the Clark committee, suggesting that 13 million Americans were suffering from hunger and malnutrition, and calling for a dramatic billion-dollar-plus program to help them.

This attempted move by OEO into food program leadership was deeply resented at the Department of Agriculture. Freeman prepared to defend his traditional territory by working up a food program that was only slightly less ambitious—one that would cost between $750 million and $1 billion and would serve nine million poor.

By this time, however, senior officers in the Budget Bureau had become concerned that competition between the two agencies would produce a report to Congress that would commit the President to a massive program at a time when Johnson was trying desperately to squeeze every dollar in a dual effort to fight inflation and finance the Vietnam war. The dispute was getting out of hand when Secretary Freeman called for White House intervention.

With Presidential Assistant Joseph Califano serving as mediator, an angry Orville Freeman and Sargent Shriver strode into the White House on July 20 to argue their plans. They were joined by Budget Bureau officials who stood ready to control any wild spending schemes they feared might break loose.

"The Office of Economic Opportunity already has shown capability for bold action on this issue," argued Shriver. "We already have helped finance the administrative cost of food programs with Operation Help, and we've set up a program to help the needy buy food stamps. . . . The same department that is helping the commercial farmer reap big profits should not also be wholly responsible for feeding the poor."

Secretary Freeman, the former three-term governor of Minnesota with a longtime liberal record, resented Shriver's slur on his department. "The improvement of food programs for the poor has always been one of my chief interests in government. That's why I took this job," contended Freeman. Arguing that it was naïve to think new food programs could be adopted without going through the agriculture committees of Congress, he insisted that only his department could deal with these committees.

White House aide Califano, listening to the two battle over the ownership of food programs, then intervened: "The President certainly isn't going to back a huge program when the proponents can't even begin to agree on how many are hungry, or where these hungry people are located." As for settling the dispute, Califano directed that "all the departments work together on a coordinated, joint response to the Clark committee."

Despite insistent prodding from Clark and Kennedy, the three departments continued their haggling, with Agriculture insisting it would not sign a report that listed more than nine million hungry persons, and OEO refusing to sign a report unless the hunger figure were placed at 13 million.

The Budget Bureau eventually had the last word. It knocked out the figure 13 million, and any language which might seem to commit the President to an action program. When they were sent the watered-down statement to sign, OEO officials conveniently lost it for a month. As a result, an equivocating, unsigned report finally was sent to the Clark committee in October—long after it might have provided momentum for further legislative action in 1967.

The report contained one valuable admission, however. The Agriculture Department recognized that the average food stamp recipient received only $200 worth of food stamps annually (using $123 of his own money to buy the stamps) while a fully adequate, low-cost diet would cost at least $345 per person. The department estimated that it would spend $330 million to aid 5.8 million persons with food stamps and commodities in fiscal 1968. A reformed program for nine million persons, providing each with a minimum diet, would cost $1.7 *billion*. By its own statistics, the Agriculture Department finally had admitted the gross failings of its food programs.

Even though the interdepartmental meetings had produced little agreement on how the Johnson Administration should respond to the Clark committee, Presidential assistant Califano ordered the same group to start working in August on another project. He directed the departments to form a Nutrition Task Force under the chairmanship of Assistant Budget Director Charles Zwick, to make recommendations for the President's 1968 legislative program and budget. Zwick's group reported privately to the White House in October, recommending a minimum $300 million increase for food programs. It called for:

- More bonus stamps "to provide all participants with an opportunity to have at least better than a 'poor diet' ";
- Uniform national eligibility standards to protect millions from exclusion from the program by state and local governments;
- Nutritional supplements for pregnant and nursing mothers and babies.

In the unlikely event that $1.5 billion were available for a program, the committee recommended it be used to start a minimum income plan, rather than to improve food programs.

For the second straight year, the President ignored his task force's recommendations.

Despite its participation in two task forces pointing up great need, the Agriculture Department asked for only a $225 million food stamp budget for fiscal 1969, barely enough to cover persons already participating and allowing no funds to bring the program up to minimum standards. In a rare reversal of roles, the Budget Bureau actually increased this request to $245 million.

Undaunted by all their setbacks, the advocates for the hungry poor began searching for another way to bring the Stennis bill to a vote in the House of Representatives. Robert Choate, who was rapidly learning the intricacies of effective lobbying, sought out Representative Albert Quie to revive Senator Stennis's emergency hunger bill. Quie, a progressive Minnesota Republican, quietly attached the emergency food aid measure as an amendment to the Economic Opportunity Act extension bill, and it sailed through Congress in November.

During the next three months, however, Choate learned that enacting a law is one thing, but persuading a reluctant administration to carry out its intent is quite another. The Johnson Administration had not requested the law, and placed a low priority on its implementation. Not until April 1968 did interdepartmental haggling finally ebb enough so that someone could begin dispensing what was supposed to be "emergency" aid to the sick and hungry poor. Five months after its enactment, this tiny emergency program finally began to send a trickle of dollars that provided at least some hungry Americans with the means to buy food stamps.

Only the needling of Choate, and of Senators Clark, Kennedy, and Javits, kept the proposed emergency program inching forward. No sooner had the three departments (USDA, HEW, and OEO) come to terms on how they would divide up the final $10 million program, than Agriculture broke the agreement. Over OEO's feeble protest, but with White House approval, Agriculture obtained $2.5 million of the limited funds for use in its overbudgeted *regular* food stamp program—the unsatisfactory program whose malfunctioning led to passage of the emergency bill in the first place!

In the final analysis, the principal 1967 legislative achievement in the battle against hunger was authorization for a national nutrition survey among the poor, to be conducted by HEW. When the Surgeon General of the United States told the poverty subcommittee in July 1967 that no one knew the extent of hunger in the nation and that no one was responsible for finding out, Javits and Kennedy, realizing the absolute necessity for official documentation of hunger in America, quietly amended another health bill to provide for the survey.

Despite the two legislative victories, no one could be very proud of the reform accomplishments of 1967 *. The emergency hunger bill finally helped a few of the poor buy food stamps and the national nutrition survey would prove helpful when results started coming in. Freeman's

---

* A chance cocktail party conversation between Senator Kennedy and CBS television producer Don Hewitt later would prove to be another important 1967 event in the politics of hunger. Kennedy convinced Hewitt that the hunger story deserved serious television exploration, thereby setting in motion a year of work on what would be a most important TV documentary.

82

reduction of food stamp prices to the poorest of the poor helped some get food, *but the winter of 1967–1968 found most of the hungry poor just as desperate as they had been a year earlier.*

"None of us covered ourselves with glory," said one participant in the Presidential task force, whose modest recommendations were ignored by the President. "With budget restrictions and disagreements between departments, we were not very bold. Agriculture had just gone through one fight with Poage and Whitten over continuing the food stamp plan, and they barely won it. They just didn't want to take them on again the next year. The President was a limiting factor, too, but Whitten still was very much in the driver's seat."

Jamie Whitten's name was not exactly a household word, and his function was not known even to veteran Washington politicians uninterested in the workings of the Agriculture Department. Even Senators Clark, Kennedy, and Javits were not aware of the extent of the Mississippi congressman's power.

But Jamie Whitten was interested in their national nutrition survey, they soon found out, and in any other matter that pertained to his department.

# CHAPTER VI

# The Subcommittee Chairman— Politics of Fear

*"What are you afraid of in Mississippi?"*

(Senator Jacob Javits to Agriculture
Secretary Orville Freeman, Senate
Poverty Subcommittee hearing on
hunger, July 1967)

WITH THE SENSITIVE INSTINCTS OF A SUCCESSFUL career bureaucrat, Dr. George Irving scanned the list of states scheduled for the National Nutrition Survey. Halfway down the column his glance froze, and he quickly dialed Congressman Jamie Whitten, the man known in Washington as the "permanent secretary of agriculture."

"Mr. Chairman, they've got Mississippi on that malnutrition study list, and I thought you'd want to know about it," dutifully reported Irving, director of the Agriculture Department's Research Service.

For the better part of 18 years as chairman of the House Appropriations Subcommittee on Agriculture, dapper Jamie L. Whitten has held an iron hand over the Department of Agriculture's budget. The entire 107,000-man department is tuned in to the Mississippi legislator's every whim.

"George, we're not going to have another smear campaign against Mississippi, are we," declared Whitten to his informant. "You boys should be thinking about a *national* survey—and do some studies in Watts and Hough and Harlem!"

Dr. Irving alerted the government's food aid network. "Mr. Whitten wants Mississippi taken off that list," he told Department of Agriculture food administrator Rodney Leonard.

Leonard, in turn, called Dr. George Silver, a Deputy Assistant Secretary of Health, Education, and Welfare, who was responsible for the joint USDA-HEW malnutrition survey.

"Jamie Whitten's found out Mississippi is on the list and is raising hell. I think we'd better drop it," Leonard said.

Silver, recalling HEW Secretary Wilbur Cohen's order to "avoid unnecessary political friction" in choosing the sample states for the hunger survey, called Dr. Arnold Schaefer, the project chief.

"Mississippi's out—politics!" Silver said curtly.

Back at the Department of Agriculture, food administrator Leonard snapped at Jamie Whitten's informant, "You couldn't have killed the project any better if you had planned it!"

Thus, in August 1967, the Johnson Administration's first meaningful attempt to ascertain the facts about hunger in Mississippi was stopped cold by an executive department's fear of one congressman. This kind of bureaucratic-congressional maneuvering, exercised between the lines of law, is little understood, seldom given public scrutiny, and far too infrequently challenged. In the quiet process of hidden power, a bureaucrat in the Agriculture Department reacts more quickly to a raised eyebrow from

85

Jamie Whitten than to a direct order from the Secretary himself. Time after time, a few words from Jamie Whitten can harden into gospel at the Department of Agriculture. Indeed, a casual Whitten statement may be so magnified as it is whispered from official to official that the response is more subservient than even the congressman had in mind.

The stocky, 59-year-old congressman is not shy about his meteoric rise from a country store in Tallahatchie County to a key position in the nation's capital. And his record is impressive—trial lawyer and state legislator at 21, district attorney for five counties at 23, U.S. congressman at 31 (in 1941), and Chairman of the Appropriations Subcommittee at 36. His steely self-confidence, studied informality, and carefully conservative clothes suggest anything but the stereotype of country-lawyer-come-to-Washington. Only the beginning of a paunch detracts from a physical sense of strength and energy that radiates from Jamie Whitten.

For all his dynamic presence, Whitten has a way of confounding a listener—or potential critic—with silky southern rhetoric. It is a test of mental agility to remember the original course of a conversation, as one high USDA official noted: "When you check on things with him, Whitten can go all around the barn with you. Oftentimes you don't fully understand what he meant. So you latch onto the most obvious point you can find and act on that."

With his implicit power, Whitten doesn't *have* to threaten or be specific. In fact, as Agriculture research official George Irving pointed out about his conversation with the congressmen that led to dropping Mississippi from the national hunger survey, "He wasn't saying 'don't go to Mississippi,' he was just suggesting that we think about other places."

Bureaucratic officials who are familiar with Whitten's oblique way of expressing his ideas know also that the Mississippian can rattle off complicated economic statistics and arguments with precise logic and organized thought.

Whitten legally holds the power of the purse, and he exercises it shrewdly. His Appropriations Subcommittee doles out funds for every item in the department's seven billion dollar budget, and it does not take long for Washington bureaucrats to realize that the chairman's wrath can destroy precious projects and throw hundreds of people out of jobs.

"He's got the most phenomenal information and total recall," one Agriculture official says of Whitten. "Once you fully understand his do's and don'ts and establish rapport with him, life is a whole lot easier!"

Jamie Whitten's considerable power is enhanced by his scholarship. He is a conscientious student of every line of the Agriculture budget, and his hawk-eye is legendary among department officials. They, in turn, anticipate his scrutiny by checking planned moves with him, thus extending to him a virtual veto on the most minute details. "A suggestion, that's all you have to have in this business," admitted Rodney Leonard.

The key to this phenomenal power—which goes beyond that of budget control—lies in Whitten's network of informants within the department, and his skill in directing their activities and operations. Executive branch officials learn to protect their own jobs, adjusting their loyalties to the legislative branch in a way the Founding Fathers may not have envisioned when they devised their splendid system of checks and balances. Bureaucratic allies of a particular congressman may be able to inject that congressman's political views (or their own) into laws or programs sponsored by an administration without the consent, or even the knowledge, of the department head. Secretaries of Agriculture may come and go, but Jamie Whitten remains, a product of Mississippi's political oligarchy and the seniority system in Congress.

Even the Secretary himself feels he must bend to the power of the "permanent Secretary." When a delegation headed by Richard Boone of the Citizens' Crusade Against Poverty had asked Orville Freeman to provide free stamps and commodities to help the hungry in Mississippi, the Secretary told them: "I've got to get along with two people in Washington—the President and Jamie Whitten. How can you help me with Whitten?"

In theory, an appropriations subcommittee only considers requests for funds to finance programs already approved by Congress. In actuality, a skillful chairman such as Whitten can control policy, alter the original authorizing legislation, and wind up virtually controlling the administration of a department.

In addition to Chairman Whitten, the Agriculture Appropriations Subcommittee has seven members: Democrats William H. Natcher of Kentucky, W. R. Hull, Jr., of Missouri, George Shipley of Illinois, and Frank Evans of Colorado; and Republicans Odin Langen of Minnesota, Robert H. Michael of Illinois, and Jack Edwards of Alabama. Because a majority of these members share Whitten's outlook on agriculture and his arch-conservative view of social action, the chairman's will becomes subcommittee's will. As chairman, he also has a hold over staff appointments.

Much of Whitten's power derives from the system within the House of Representatives. Once a subcommittee makes a decision, the full House Appropriations Committee almost always backs it up. This is particularly true with agriculture appropriations, because House Appropriations Chairman George Mahon of Texas shares Whitten's views on farm policy, welfare spending, and racial issues. For years, Whitten has been in absolute control of all bills before his subcommittee, from the first markup session to the final House vote. "The lines in my face would be deeper except for you," Mahon inscribed his own portrait in the Mississippian's office.

The House at large rarely has challenged Agriculture budgets because most nonfarm bloc members find the subject too complex or dull, and rarely take the trouble to inform themselves about it. If some members, or the public, are roused to the point where a challenge develops, the House's committee chairmen generally pull together to defeat the move. Committee members follow to insure that they will have the chairman's support for their own pet bills—and to keep sacrosanct the whole system of mutual support and protection.

If a challenge happens to get out of hand, the first commandment of a subcommittee chairman is, "Never let yourself in for a battle on the House floor if there is any chance for defeat." Part of the power of a chairman stems from his apparent invincibility—and the image must be preserved! (Therefore, Whitten went along with the Nixon Administration's full budget request for food aid in 1969, knowing there was sufficient pressure for a much bigger appropriation. Whitten responded here only to the politics of the issue, not the substance, for he still complained to Senator George McGovern that hunger was not a problem, that "Nigras won't work" if you give them free food, and that McGovern was promoting revolution by continuing to seek free food stamps for the poorest Americans.)

Where agriculture legislation is concerned, Whitten must share power to some measure with Senator Spessard

Holland, a Florida Democrat who chairs the Senate Appropriations Subcommittee on Agriculture. Holland is a blunt man who insists that Section 32 funds—food dollars from customs receipts—should be held in reserve to be used at the proper time to boost the prices of his state's citrus, vegetable, and beef industries. Thus, when Whitten and Holland act in unison—as they often do—the results are predictable. After the School Lunch Act was liberalized in 1964, they managed to refuse funding free school lunches for more than two years. The Johnson Administration had sought only two or three million dollars to help some of the estimated five million poor children who got no benefits from the lunch program, but all the funds were held back in committee until Senator Philip Hart of Michigan threatened to take the fight to the floor.

Jamie Whitten's power is greater than Holland's, however, not only because appropriations usually originate in the House, but also because in the smaller body of the Senate (contrary to its reputation, the Senate is now the more liberal, flexible body), there is less hesitation to overturn subcommittee decisions than in the tradition-bound House of Representatives. The House system, therefore, assures more *inherent* power for its subcommittee chairmen, and Jamie Whitten has been vigorous and skillful in pursuing it.

Just back from their discovery of hunger in Mississippi in April 1967, Dr. Robert Coles and the three other Field Foundation doctors found out about Whitten's influence when they appealed to Orville Freeman. They walked into the Secretary's office feeling that they would be welcomed as helpful, authoritative reporters of the facts, and they left feeling that they had been tagged as troublemakers.

"We were told that we and all the hungry children we

had examined and all the other hungry Americans . . . would have to reckon with Mr. Jamie L. Whitten, as indeed must the Secretary of Agriculture, whose funds come to him through the kindness of the same Mr. Whitten. We were told of the problems that the Agriculture Department has with Congress, and we left feeling we ought to weigh those problems as somehow of the same order as the problems we had met in the South—and that we know from our work elsewhere existed all over the country," recalled Coles.

When Senator Jacob Javits asked Agriculture Secretary Freeman, "What are you afraid of in Mississippi?" (at the July 1967 hearing on hunger in Mississippi) the New York liberal wanted to know why Freeman would not modify the food program to reach more of the hungry in Mississippi and elsewhere. The only response he got was ex-Marine Freeman's outthrust jaw and a growl that he was not afraid of anyone and would not be intimidated.

Nevertheless, faced with Jamie Whitten's power over his department, and fed information by a Whitten-conscious bureaucracy, Freeman had failed for two years to take measures to feed more of the hungry poor in America. Moreover, the Secretary had stubbornly refused to acknowledge the chasm between his department's efforts and the real needs of the hungry.

From Freeman on down, every Agriculture Department official knew that hunger spelled "hound dog" to Jamie Whitten.

"You've got to understand how Jamie feels about 'hound dog' projects," a career official explained. (In southern country jargon, a "hound dog" is always hanging around, useless, waiting to be thrown scraps.) Years before, the chairman had killed a small pilot project to teach unemployed southern Negroes how to drive tractors. "Now, that's a 'hound dog' project, and I don't want to see any more of them," he had said.

Whitten's opposition to any program resembling social welfare—or aid to Negroes—contributed to the failure of War on Poverty programs for rural America. When President Johnson signed an executive order giving the Agriculture Department responsibility for coordinating the rural war on poverty, Secretary Freeman created a Rural Development Service to give the Department a focal point for helping the poor. It was designed to coordinate programs meeting all the needs of the rural poor—housing, education, water, food—not only within the Agriculture Department, but throughout the federal government.

Within a year, the Rural Community Development Service was dead. "Whitten thought the Service smacked of social experimentation and civil rights," a Department of Agriculture official said. In addition, Whitten's brother-in-law, one of many cronies who have filled Agriculture jobs over the years, had clashed with Robert G. Lewis, the idealistic Wisconsin progressive who headed the program. Whitten simply cut off the funds, and pigeonholed the coordinating powers of RCDS by placing the responsibility with the docile, conservative Farmers' Home Administration. Freeman never fought the issue. There were too many other essential matters, other appropriations, that were more important to him, so the embryonic effort to coordinate rural poverty programs through the Department of Agriculture ended as little more than a passing idea.

(By assigning the broad rural poverty responsibility to the Department of Agriculture, President Johnson, like President Nixon after him, indicated either a great naïveté about the Department or a lack of seriousness in his proposals. The four congressional committees with which the

92

Department of Agriculture must deal undoubtedly are the least receptive of any in Congress to provide meaningful help to the hardcore rural poor.)

Jamie Whitten has wielded that kind of influence since the mid-1940s, when he killed an emerging Agriculture Department study which tried to anticipate the social and economic problems of Negro GI's returning from World War II to the feudal cotton South. At that time, the Mississippi congressman was the youngest chairman of an appropriations subcommittee. By opposing all studies exploring the effects of a changing agriculture upon people, Whitten helped insure that Agriculture Department farm policy would never seriously include consideration of the effects of its programs on sharecroppers or farm workers. Whitten and the other equally powerful southern congressmen who share his views insured that the Department of Agriculture would focus only on the cotton planter and his crop. As a result, farm policies which have consistently ignored their toll on millions of black poor have contributed to a rural-urban migration, to a civil rights revolution, and to the ruin of many Americans.

With his wily ability to juggle figures and cloud ideas, Whitten has convinced officials unfamiliar with his technique (and lacking intimate knowledge of the facts) that he is quite a reasonable man—especially when the conversation turns to hunger and the food programs. As he tells it, he was a pioneer on the nutrition issue.

In 1950, he fought for funds for a Department of Agriculture cook book, and he warned the House it had better concern itself with human as well as animal health. To this day, Whitten insists that the Agriculture Department keep the book in print; he sends a free copy to newlyweds in his district.

The Subcommittee Chairman also denies that he paralyzed Freeman on the hunger issue: "I *helped* the Secretary by making two points with him," Whitten insists. "I told him he had to charge people what they were accustomed to paying for food stamps because that's what the law says. . . . And I pointed out to him that the law forbids selling food stamps and distributing commodities in the same counties." By making these two helpful points, Whitten blocked the most feasible emergency measures.

"Why, I gave him more money for those food programs than he could spend!" said Whitten.

Actually, the hopelessly inadequate $45 million for food programs Whitten "gave" to Freeman were fought, bought, and paid for by the administration and congressional liberals; this was what was left after Whitten and Holland whittled down the original $100 million, three-year authorization won by liberals on the House floor.

Whitten's explanations of food programs may have appeared perfectly reasonable to Freeman, Sargent Shriver, and many members of Congress, but their total impact was to stop any reform that would get food to the hungry. His own strongly held view is that the food programs should serve the farm programs, not vice versa, and his actions over the years have halted any kind of aid the Agriculture Department might have directed toward the poor. In the early 1960s, when the Kennedy Administration was momentarily concerned for the poor of Appalachia, the Department of Agriculture found a way to provide housing grants to aid the hardest-core poor, but once Whitten discovered the grant program in operation, he killed all further appropriations for it.

A few years later, a new cotton program provided advance payments to cotton farmers for withdrawing some of their acreage from production. Sharecroppers, who provided most of the cotton labor force, were supposed to receive their "share" of government payments for idle land. With Whitten's inspiration or blessing, the Department of Agriculture adopted a regulation permitting the plantation owner to deduct from the sharecropper's government payments the amount he claimed was owed for the sharecropper's rent, farming expnses, etc. Under the feudal system, however, the sharecropper *never* had any legal guarantee that he would receive his fair share of profit for the crop he produced. Blacks who declined to turn over their checks were kicked off hundreds of plantations. The Agriculture Department did not halt the practice.

One of Whitten's sharecropper constituents, trying desperately to find food for her family, gave her own intuitive view of her congressman's attitudes: "He's probably with the bossman's side, don't you know. He's with them. No one's with us but ourselves, and no matter how many of us there are, we don't have what they have."

Although much of the legislation he favors has enriched American agriculture business with government funds, Whitten's stock answer to any liberalization of the Department of Agriculture food programs is that they are "food programs, not welfare programs." He is adamant about suggestions that food programs be moved to the more liberal Department of Health, Education, and Welfare. "Who'll see to it that [funds for food] don't go for frivolity and wine?" he asks.

Whitten's views on welfare, so strongly felt through the Department of Agriculture, are shared by many Americans. Yet when viewed against the background of Tallahatchie County and its social history, these views, and their interpretations through Agriculture Department programs, take on a different meaning. Since hunger means poverty, and poverty, in Mississippi, usually means black, any expanded aid to the hungry means one more threat to the socioeconomic order in which the black worker has always been held in absolute dependency upon crumbs from the plantation owner.

The 100,000 or more black Mississippi farm workers who suddenly found themselves with nothing to hold onto in the winter of 1967 were little concerned with frivolity and wine. They had lost their sole supply of food, as Mississippi counties switched over from the inadequate but free surplus commodities to a food stamp program the poor could not afford. "No work, no money, and now, no food," was their outcry, and they desperately sought a reduction in the price of stamps at the very moment when Jamie Whitten was starting his annual review of the Department of Agriculture's budget, with its accompanying discourse on the nature of the poor man. He had heard, the Chairman said, that "organized groups" sought to make food stamps free to the poor.

"This is one of the things you always run into," he said to Secretary Freeman. "You make stamps available at 30 percent discount; then they want them at 50, then 75. Now, I have heard reports that some of the organized minority groups are insisting they be provided free of charge. . . . When you start giving people something for nothing, just giving them all they want for nothing, I wonder if you don't destroy character more than you might improve nutrition. I think more and more American people are coming to that conclusion."

They built a lot of character in Mississippi that winter, where the disruption caused by the abrupt changeover to food stamps contributed to the kind of wholesale destitution not seen in this country since the Great Depression.

But the Chairman did not seem to think his black constituents were learning the character lesson well enough when it came to the school lunch and new school breakfast programs. Out of work and out of money, few Mississippi Negroes could afford to give their children 25 cents a day for a school lunch, and few schools provided the free lunches which the law technically required for the poor. Department of Agriculture officials virtually begged that the special school lunch assistance budget be raised from two million to ten million dollars annually to give meals to an added 360,000 children in poor areas. Whitten expressed concern only about the impact of civil rights sanctions as he slashed the request by two-thirds.

When another project—a requested million dollars for a pilot school breakfast program to help the neediest youngsters—came up, Whitten's patience wore thin. "Do you contemplate having a pilot dinner program—evening meals—called supper where I grew up?" Whitten asked sarcastically.

When Agriculture Department officials explained that "a hungry child in the morning is not able to take full advantage of the schooling that is offered," Whitten wanted to know why the government should be supplying what the family should have supplied before they left home.

"We all recognize that the type of home from which some children come affects them in many, many ways, but there is a problem always as to whether the federal government should start doing everything for the citizens. You may end up with a certain class of people doing nothing to help themselves. To strike a happy medium is always a real problem."

In this case, Whitten struck it by cutting all $6.5 million requested for breakfast funds from the budget.

Each time a group of doctors, team of reporters, or other investigation produced firsthand reports of hunger

97

in the South, Whitten launched his own "investigation" and announced that parental neglect is largely responsible for any problems. In 1968, when the drive for a bigger food program began to gather steam nationally, Whitten sent out the FBI to disprove the existence of the problem.

The Mississippi congressman demands that the poor, if they are to get any benefits, must prove they are hungry on a case-by-case basis. "These doctors . . . have not submitted any names . . . ," he wrote one concerned northern lady, assuring her that he would be "most sympathetic and helpful in trying to work this matter out."

Time after time, Whitten has requested names and addresses of the poor who complain of ill-treatment in his home state. Yet in Jamie Whitten's home county the thought of having their names known strikes terror among those who have had dealing with the local officials.

A news team from television's Public Broadcast Laboratory, interviewing a black housewife in Whitten's home town of Charleston, felt the danger involved in "naming names." As Mrs. Metcalf began to explain why the food stamp and school lunch programs were not helping her family, a task force of sedans and panel trucks began to cruise back and forth on the U.S. highway about 50 yards from her plantation shack. Suddenly the trucks lunged off the highway into the shack's front yard, surrounding the television crew's two station wagons. A rifle or shotgun was mounted in the rear window of each truck.

"You're trespassing. Git!" growled the plantation manager as he pushed his way past the TV reporter and ordered Mrs. Metcalf to get outside the shack if she knew what was good for her.

"You were trespassing when you crossed the Mississippi state line," shouted Deputy Sheriff Buck Shaw as he ordered the PBL crew to clear out.

In an attempt to insure Mrs. Metcalf's safety from the local "law," the reporter phoned Congressman Whitten in Washington.

"You remember when Martin Luther King went through my town?" the congressman answered. "You read the *Wall Street Journal?* It said that he went through there and everybody turned out to look at him. And as soon as he left, they just turned over and went back to sleep. . . . I just know, I live down there and I know. . . . Good God, Chicago, Washington, Detroit . . . every one of them would give any amount of money if they could go to sleep feeling as safe—both races—as my folks will!"

It wasn't so peaceful about three o'clock that afternoon with those hard-eyed men threatening Mrs. Metcalf, the reporter explained.

"I suspect Deputy Shaw's like I am," Whitten snapped. "They recognized when you crossed that state line you had no good intention in your mind. I'm no kingfish. I just know my people and my people get along. Unfortunately, you folks and the folks up here don't know how to get along. . . . I bet you money if I ran tomorrow, and nobody voted except the colored people, I'd get the majority. I grew up where five or six of my closest neighbors were Negroes. We played together as kids. We swapped vegetables. Why, I grew up hugging my Momma, and my Momma hugging them."

There were as many Negroes as whites at his father's funeral, Whitten asserts—and he keeps on his desk a yellowed 1936 newspaper editorial that praised District Attorney Jamie Whitten for successfully prosecuting the white man who burned some Mississippi Negroes to death.

Against Whitten's statements about how he is respected by Negroes and would get their vote, about how close his

99

relationship and understanding with Negroes has been, about how quiet and peaceful life is in Charleston, another point of view appeared, as one of his black constituents spoke on the same subject—rambling much as Jamie Whitten does. An eloquent, middle-aged woman told Dr. Robert Coles about the plantation owner for whom her husband works, about his wife, about food, and about life in America:

"He [the plantation owner] doesn't want us trying to vote and like that—and first I'd like to feed my kids, before I go trying to vote.

"His wife—the boss man's—she'll come over here sometimes give me some extra grits and once or twice in the year some good bacon. She tells me we get along fine down here and I says 'yes' to her. What else would I be saying, I ask you?

"But it's no good. The kids aren't eating enough, and you'd have to be wrong in the head, pure crazy to say they are. Sometimes we talk of leaving; but you know it's just no good up there either, we hear. They eat better, but they have bad things up there I hear, rats as big as raccoons, I hear, and they bit my sister's kid real bad.

"It's no kind of country to be proud of, with all this going on—the colored people still having it so bad, and the kids being sick and there's nothing you can do about it." *

Whitten's affection for black constituents like this woman does not extend to federal measures to assist their lot in life. Of the 24,081 residents of Tallahatchie County, 18,000 have family incomes less than $3,000 a year, and 15,197 make less than $2,000. Of these thousands legally defined as poor, only 2,367 qualify for public assistance,

* Robert Coles and Harry Huge, "We Need Help," *The New Republic*, March 8, 1969, p. 20.

and 6,710 receive food stamps. Only a few blocks from Whitten's own white frame house, Negroes live in shacks without toilets, running water, electricity—or food.

Whitten and his fellow white Mississippians point with great pride to the economic progress their state has made in recent years. Improved farming methods, conversion of marginal cropland to timber and other uses, and a strong soil bank program have greatly enriched the commercial farmer in Mississippi. Other government prorams, including state tax inducements, have promoted wide industrialization, and rural white workers have found new affluence in the hundreds of factories and small shops that have sprung up.

But the new farming has eliminated thousands of jobs for Negro plantation workers while the segregated social system denies them factory jobs. The able-bodied usually head north, leaving the very young, the very old, and the unskilled to cope with progress. The rural black does not share in the new prosperity of Mississippi, and some Negroes are "worse off" than at any time since the Depression. Indeed, in many parts of the Deep South the black man is literally being starved out by the new prosperity.

Perhaps the white southern politician is no more to blame than are whites anywhere. But the white in the South could not afford to see the truth of the Negro's suffering because to feel that truth would have shattered a whole way of life.

Jamie Whitten truly believes in his own fairness, his idea of good works, and the imagined affection he receives from Negroes back home. For 59 years, he has anesthetized his soul to the human misery and indignity only a few yards from his own home, and has refused to believe that the responsibility for that indignity lies on his white shoulders. His belief in the basic laziness, indifference, and unworthiness of the black poor is as strong as his belief in the virtues of a way of life that for three centuries has denied these same black poor any avenues of pursuing ambition, self-respect, or a better future for their children.

That Jamie Whitten should suffer from blindness to human need is one thing. But that he can use his blindness as an excuse to limit the destiny of millions of Americans is another matter, one which should concern anyone who believes in the basic strengths of this country's constitutional guarantees. The checks and balances of a reasonable democratic republic have gone completely awry when a huge bureaucracy and the top officials of an administration base their actions concerning deepest human need on their fearful perception of what one rather limited man seems to want.

The system of seniority and temerity that gives a man such as Jamie Whitten such awesome power must come under more serious public scrutiny if the American system of government is ever to establish itself on the basis of moral concern about the individual human being.

# CHAPTER VII

# The Politics of Ignorance

IF JAMIE WHITTEN SUFFERED A STRANGE IGNO-
rance about the desperate straits of his poor neighbors, he
had plenty of company.

As soon as the hunger issue surfaced in 1967, politicians, scientists, and private citizens tangled in an angry,
inconclusive debate that ostensibly concerned the nature of hunger, but in its full depth raised doubts about
the nature of American society.

It started with a simple question: Are the poor in
America hungry?

Robert Kennedy, Dr. Robert Coles, and others who
actually visited the poor answered, "Yes," but most local
officials denied the existence of hunger in their areas.

As the Senate Poverty Subcommittee and the Citizens'
Board of Inquiry continued to accumulate evidence, local
politicians and opponents of food aid reform changed

their stance. If the poor are hungry, they said, it is because they are ignorant about proper nutrition. The experts who were brought in disagreed among themselves about whether lack of knowledge or lack of money was responsible. As the Citizens' Board of Inquiry conducted more interviews, its members became convinced that little was known about all aspects of hunger in the United States. This led to still another question: Why don't we know?

One comforting answer was that we don't know because hunger and malnutrition are no longer serious problems. But there was a more disturbing answer: We don't know because we have not looked; we have not looked because we feared what we would see; and we were afraid because seeing would indict us.

If this theory were true, then America's ignorance about poverty and hunger did not happen by accident. Instead, self-interest, greed, indifference, and a deep self-deception combined to soothe the man of conscience and permit his personal ethic to function smoothly. This theory implies that we, not the poor, suffered from ignorance.

Following their Mississippi trip, Senators Kennedy and Clark badgered the government for statistics and evaluations of the nutritional health of low-income Americans, but they received no answers. Finally a barrage of questions from Clark at the subcommittee's July 1967 hearings produced a startling admission from the government's top physicians.

"We do not know the extent of malnutrition anywhere in the United States," said the Surgeon General of the U.S. Public Health Service, William H. Stewart.

"Whose job is it to find out?" asked Senator Clark.

"That's part of the problem," Dr. Stewart replied. "It

hasn't been anybody's job. We can do it all over the world, but not in the United States."

Despite Dr. Stewart's admission of ignorance, many government officials continued to dismiss the possibility that millions of people lacked adequate nutrition in the richest nation in the history of the world.

For 2½ years the highest elected and appointed officials in the United States Government debated the nature and scope of hunger. Emergency aid was delayed while the government argued over numbers of poor, the causes of malnutrition, and the motives of the men who originally raised the hunger issue. As the debate wore on, it became obvious that affluent America was far more ignorant about its poor citizens than the poor were ignorant about nutrition.

Meanwhile, the Citizens' Board of Inquiry listened to another kind of argument—concerning the right of the poor to survive in America. Debates about budget priorities, welfare philosophies, and political motives faded as the investigators moved out from Washington into the country where the poor told their own stories—stories of human suffering that added up to a bitter indictment of the nation's welfare system.

Dr. Vivian Henderson, a Board of Inquiry member and president of Clark College in Atlanta, conducted his first hearing in San Antonio, a city with 150,000 poor Mexican-Americans. As story after story of hunger and ill treatment spilled out before the Board, a young mother, too timid to speak, handed Chairman Henderson a piece of paper.

The Negro educator sat silent in the Santa Cruz chapel reading the crudely scrawled note. Finally, he said softly, "I don't want to comment because I'll curse."

The young mother had written that she had just left the hearing to go home for lunch, where she found a notice from the city saying that her family of 11 would be evicted from the public housing quarter if $10 in back rent were not paid by five o'clock that afternoon. Mrs. Frances Delgado testified that her family had little to eat and could not qualify for welfare because her unemployed husband was considered able to work. An employment service official then explained that *there are 22 unskilled laborers like Delgado for every one unskilled job in San Antonio.*

Physicians gave a further dimension to the problems of Mexican-Americans in this charming southwestern city. "I have seen children at the Robert B. Green Hospital three, four, and five years old, who weighed only 20 pounds. I know of at least 10 children who came to us at the age of two to four months, and all of them weighed no more than they had at birth," testified Dr. Charles B. Hilton, a physician highly respected in the community.

Vera Burke, Director of Social Services for the county charity hospital, explained further that expectant mothers usually are so anemic that they are given blood transfusions as a matter of routine before delivery. "We see malnourished babies a year old weighing seven pounds. We see the results of this kind of malnutrition in mental retardation. We see patients with diabetes who are unable to buy the necessary food to comply with the dietary requirements. It seems to me," she said angrily, "that it is bad economy to pay for medical care rather than provide the necessities of life that would eliminate the need for it!" The horror of the San Antonio hearing was repeated in Birmingham and Boston, New York City and Appalachia.

On a field trip through New York City's black ghetto areas, Citizens' Board of Inquiry members heard Dr. Harold Wise describe the malnutrition cases—especially

106

among children—that come into the Bronx's Montefiore Hospital. "The most common cause of 'failure to thrive' cases in infants here is insufficient calorie intake," said Montefiore pediatrician Laurance Feinberg.

In Appalachia, the Board of Inquiry found that hunger is no respecter of skin color. In Hazard, Kentucky, the faces in the Union Hall were mostly white, but the stories were the same. Board members Dr. James Carter, professor of nutrition at Vanderbilt University, questioned Mrs. Lily Ivory, who said she could not afford the $48 a month lump sum payment required to participate in the food stamp program.

"Your children are between the ages of two and twelve. Do they have milk every day?" he asked.

"No. . . . I get milk once a month when my check comes in and they only have it one day and that's all."

"And meat?"

"They usually have it on Fridays and Sunday."

"Would you say that your children complain of hunger?"

"All the time."

Even where there are stamps, they seldom provide enough food, the Board found. "You can't make it nohow on the food stamps," said Sherman Nease, an unemployed miner with nine children. "Last part of the second week it starts running out. Then you use credit. But my credit has run out, too."

Board of Inquiry member Harry Huge (pronounced Hew'-ghy), a District of Columbia attorney, and staff member David Hearne found Florida's west coast alive with affluent vacationers who provided a stark contrast to the impoverished Negros in the slums of Fort Myers and the migrant fruit pickers in the camp at Immokalee. They saw so many pale and sickly children in one afternoon that, although neither investigator is a physician, they sent 23 migrant youngsters to Variety Children's Hospital in Miami. The hospital reported 39 serious illnesses among the 23 children.

In Boston, Hearne and Board member Dr. Raymond Wheeler were told by a young resident doctor at Boston City Hospital that "the major cause of infant deaths here is pneumonia—no longer an important killer except in the weak, malnourished, and chronically ill."

For nine months, the Board of Inquiry toured the forgotten corners of this country, holding hearings and collecting the poignant human evidence of the extent of deprivation. At the same time, the Board's staff members in Washington started asking some hard questions of American medicine, and more American ignorance was documented.

From Harvard and Yale, Cornell and Columbia, Vanderbilt and Baylor, the experts all said they knew more about the nutritional status of persons in 31 underdeveloped countries of the world than of Americans, rich or poor. These scientists and professors of nutrition had been recruited by the government in 1955 to perform studies for the Interdepartmental Committee on Nutrition for National Defense, a cooperative effort involving the State Department and its Agency for International Development, along with the Departments of Defense, Agriculture, and Health, Education, and Welfare. It was considered in the national interest "to deal with nutrition problems of technical, military, and economic importance" in these foreign countries where the government hoped to deter the spread of communism. In the United States itself, the group studied only the nutritional status of two Indian reservations—and found hunger and misery, which went unnoticed and untreated.

The Board of Inquiry learned not only that American medicine has not studied malnutrition in this country, but also that the American doctor is poorly prepared to deal with it in his own practice. "Clinical nutrition is not even taught in most medical schools and is not really adequately done in any of them," commented Dr. Nevin Scrimshaw, head of the Department of Nutrition and Food Science at Massachusetts Institute of Technology.

"Most physicians are not well trained to identify malnutrition except for gross underweight or overweight, and this anyone can do," said Dr. Frederick J. Stare, chairman of the Department of Nutrition at the Harvard University Medical School. Dr. Stare blamed the economics of medical research for ignorance about the nutritional health of the poor. "Nobody has put up the money," he said. "You have to do the work where you can get the money." The money had been forthcoming only for research on diseases of the rich, the problems of the farmer who wanted to get more eggs out of his chicken with less feed, and the problems of the military, which wanted the underdeveloped countries to become strong enough to resist communism.

A member of the Board of Inquiry, Dr. M. Alfred Haynes, associate professor at the Johns Hopkins School of Hygiene and Public Health, believed that more than economics is involved. "Medical education," he said, "is often obsessed with the acute, the dramatic, and the esoteric. Medical students know far more about rare, inborn errors of metabolism which they may see once in a lifetime than they do about the problems of hunger in their immediate vicinity. . . . We have ignored the problem of malnutrition because we did not know it existed. We did not know it existed because we did not look for it. We did not look for it because it was embarrassing for us to think about it as existing in our own country. . . ."

If the university researcher had to depend on outside funds for his projects, the federal government certainly did not. Yet the various bureaus in Health, Education, and Welfare spent millions on nutritional research, again without devoting any attention to the health of the poor. Surgeon General Stewart offered his own theory about this strange ignorance within the supposedly finest medical system in the world:

"Somehow a glass curtain has descended around the best in American medicine. On one side of the curtain is the gleaming, antiseptic world of medical excellence. Its wonders are plainly visible to those outside. But admission is by ticket only, and the line to the box office stretches out of sight. For a time it seemed that the curtain was made of one-way glass. People outside could see in, but those inside scarcely seemed to notice the faces against the pane."

As the Citizens' Board of Inquiry Washington research staff studied medical school, state board of health, and public health service data on malnutrition, they found that individual American doctors have been reporting the occurrence of a high percentage of iron deficiency anemia among pregnant women and children of poverty for more than 40 years, yet the condition has never been dealt with decisively. The Board of Inquiry discovered that no state department of health kept statistics on incidence of malnutrition, and only about 50 medical nutritionists practiced the science in all of state government. Over 30 years ago, during an exciting period of social research, the Agriculture Department had studied the diets of the poor, but it then deserted the subject except for national food consumption surveys every ten years—surveys *which should have prompted emergency nutrition research.* Led by the Rockefeller and Ford Foundations, the private foundations studied nutrition in India, as did the food industry's Agribusiness Council, but each turned down requests to help improve nutrition of poor Americans. Of all the private United Fund organizations, only the Cleveland charity supported a major effort to study the nutritional needs of the American poor.

On April 22, 1968, more than a hundred reporters gathered at the famous old Willard Hotel in Washington to hear Leslie Dunbar and the Citizens' Board of Inquiry reveal the results of their study.

"We have found concrete evidence of chronic hunger and malnutrition in every part of the United States where we have held hearings or conducted field trips," Dunbar announced. He stated that at least ten million Americans suffer from hunger and malnutrition.

The Board of Inquiry report was published in a paperback book filled with pictures of human faces that reflected the ravages of hunger, and pages of documentation for every fact it presented. *Hunger USA,* as the book was titled, delivered a searing indictment of the Agriculture Department, the Agriculture and Appropriations Committees of Congress, the medical and public health professions, food manufacturers, and local government—charging that all of our institutions had failed the hungry poor.

In *Hunger USA* the Board of Inquiry classified 256 counties in the United States as "hunger counties" requiring immediate emergency assistance. For a county to be so designated, three of four conditions had to be present: the percentage of poor people had to be at least twice the national average of 20 percent; the postneonatal mortality rate (deaths of infants between one month

*111*

and one year) had to be twice the national average; and the level of participation in welfare or in government food programs had to be less than 25 percent of the poor population. This formula skipped entirely the vast urban ghettoes and pockets of extreme poverty amid great affluence, and marked out mostly rural counties in the Southeast and Southwest.

The immediate roar of protest from public officials in virtually every one of the hunger counties was equaled only by the roar from the agriculture committees in Congress—whose members represented some of the earmarked "hunger counties" and at the same time held responsibility in Congress for administering the malfunctioning food programs.

Five days after the Board of Inquiry made public its findings, House Agriculture Chairman Bob Poage of Texas started his own investigation. In a letter to the county health officer in each of the 256 "emergency hunger counties," Poage gave clear hints of his own presumptions, which he wanted corroborated.

"The first indictment is that hunger and malnutrition exist in this country affecting millions of our fellow Americans and increasing in severity and extent from year to year," he wrote. "From my limited knowledge of nutrition I would assume that it was true that many Americans suffer from an improper diet, but the problem there is one of education or of personal decisions. . . ."

Five months later, Chairman Poage issued a House Agriculture Committee report, based on responses from 212 of the 256 county health officers. The report was couched in language that reflected the bombastic Texas Congressman's own feelings about the poor:

"The basic problem is one of ignorance as to what constitutes a balanced diet, coupled with indifference by a

112

great many persons who should and probably do not know . . . deliberate parental neglect . . . relief clients are virtually uneducable . . . mentally retarded parents are blamed in a great many instances for the neglect of children . . . fatherless households, with children born out of wedlock, are blamed for distressing conditions . . . children suffered because a father spent disproportionately large sums either on liquor or on extramarital sexual relations . . . jobs were available in a community but rejected by able-bodied men who apparently preferred to remain on welfare rolls . . . families on food relief often had television sets and nice automobiles, and often the head of the household was reported to be spending money on whiskey that was needed for the purchase of food for the children. . . ."

In short, Bob Poage—nonscientist, nonphysician, chairman of the committee that writes food legislation for the hungry poor—determined that any poor American who is hungry or malnourished is in that condition because of ignorance, immorality, degeneration, retardation, or cruelty.

The predominantly southern county health officers who responded to Chairman Poage's inquiry did indeed provide the Texan with answers that enforced his feelings about the unworthiness of the poor. Yet, in their replies, the doctors also made medical findings that Poage chose not to emphasize in his report. For whenever the responding doctors stopped defending their communities and trying their hands as philosophers, psychologists, economists, and political scientists, they spoke eloquently and with authority about both hunger and malnutrition. Nutritionists at the University of Iowa School of Medicine analyzed all the responses to Poage's inquiry, and decided that his committee report "produces abundant evidence that there is hunger and malnutrition in the United States," despite the completely biased and misleading manner in which Poage phrased his questions.

Behind Poage's attack on *Hunger USA* lay another concern—that farm support programs might be lost if the huge agriculture budget were to come under fire from the general public. Poage did not disguise his concern that the Board of Inquiry report would lead to heavier federal expenditures for food programs. He explained to fellow House members how much already was being spent on food programs, then added, "All of these expenditures are charged to the budget of the Department of Agriculture, and form the basis of much of the undeserved criticism of 'extravagant expenditure' on behalf of the farmers."

Once again, Chairman Poage did not tell the whole story. Of the $7 billion Department of Agriculture budget in 1968, $3 billion was paid directly to farmers in price supports. Only $340 million went to school lunch program and food stamp recipients, and $410 million went to pay farmers for commodities in the commodity program.

Poage emphasized that six million poor persons received food assistance, but he did not say that millions did not—including thousands in the 153 Texas counties without any food assistance, and more thousands in the other 101 Texas counties where only 9 percent received food aid. He stressed that two million poor children received free or reduced-price meals, but did not say that another five million children legally entitled to those free meals did not receive them. (Poage's home state recorded one of the lowest percentages of poor children receiving school lunch food aid.)

The challenge to the Citizens' Board of Inquiry report which occupied Bob Poage for five months was only beginning. While Agriculture Committee Chairman Poage conducted his mail research with county health officials, Agriculture Appropriations Subcommittee Chairman Whitten sent FBI agents all over the country to investigate what Whitten conceived as a deliberately "framed picture" in *Hunger USA* and in "Hunger in America," a powerful CBS documentary which was shown in May and perhaps more than any event in 1968 added to the demand for reform. The photos in *Hunger USA* looked suspiciously familiar, he said, reminding him of old Agriculture Department photos of poverty in faraway lands.

The FBI agents assigned to the House Appropriations Committee did not seek to investigate conditions of hunger or poverty, but systematically began to question countless persons connected in any way with the Board of Inquiry or the CBS documentary. They concentrated on items which particularly fascinated Whitten, such as the photograph of a bony, emaciated dog which appeared in *Hunger USA* over the caption, " 'Where you see a starving dog such as this one,' the doctor said, 'you'll find hungry people.' "

Pointing to page 39 in the red-white-and-blue *Hunger USA*, FBI agent Charles Wultich began questioning photographer Al Clayton about the dog.

"That's the dog in Atlanta?" asked Wultich.

"That's not Atlanta," replied Clayton. "That's Baker County, Georgia."

"You know whom that dog belonged to? Did you take it at a family's house?"

"I took it on the road," answered Clayton.

"You don't know whose dog it was?" asked the exasperated FBI agent—and so it went for more than 200 questions as agent Wultich tried to find out whether photographer Clayton really had seen the sad, misshapen black and white poor people shown in his photographs, and whether Clayton had been hired in unusual, conspiratorial fashion by the Field Foundation.

When the agent left, the photographer turned off his concealed tape recorder and telephoned Board of Inquiry member Harry Huge, an attorney who was trying to monitor Whitten's probe in order to be ready for any smear attack. Clayton chuckled at the FBI agent's comical questioning until he remembered that the agents also would be grilling the poor people shown in his pictures.

"I don't know why those being investigated got so excited," said Jamie Whitten about the protests against his FBI investigation. "They already know if their facts are right. We are just starting to find out."

For the frightened Mexican-Americans in the *barrios* of San Antonio, the important fact was that they had been visited by "two men with suits on" who asked innumerable questions about their private lives, and compared their answers—down to the most minute details—with what they had told the Board of Inquiry. A San Antonio priest, who protested that the FBI investigation was harrassing poor people who were guilty of no greater crime than petitioning their government for help, found himself under investigation for his protest.

"What do you mean by intimidation?" the new team of FBI agents asked Father Ralph Ruiz. "Any specific acts? Do you know of any force? Any aggressive behavior on their part? We're trying to find out whether there was any intimidation in the legal sense—any obstruction of justice on these people's part."

When the priest tried to explain why a poor, illiterate, half-starved, unemployed Mexican-American is intimidated by two strange FBI men who enter his house, look in his cupboards, and ask him countless questions, the agents asked what could possibly be wrong with their ascertaining the facts.

The investigation continued, involving hundreds of man-hours, because between the uneducated poor and the precise lawyers, there was no common definition of facts.

The conservative politicians of the Deep South, surrounded by 300 years of miserable black slavery and poverty, were obsessed with the idea of having anyone who contends there is suffering prove out his facts in an airtight legal case. For example, when Senators Kennedy and Clark toured Mississippi, they met an unemployed Negro who could not afford food stamps. They remembered him well because of his name and the zestful exchange in which the man had said "So you're Robert Kennedy," and Kennedy had laughed, "So you're Andrew Jackson!" At a hearing, after Clark cited Jackson's problems as an example, Mississippi Senator Stennis made a long distance telephone call and then reported that the sheriff, "a very responsible young man," cannot find an Andrew Jackson in Cleveland, Mississippi.

Clark had made a mistake in that Andrew Jackson lived in a small town adjoining Cleveland. It is not likely that Senator Stennis, with hungry Negroes living within several hundred yards of his home in DeKalb, really doubted the existence of the Andrew Jacksons of his state. He was merely making a good lawyer's best defense for a client he knows is guilty.

At the same time that Congressmen Whitten and Poage were investigating the Citizens' Board of Inquiry and its report, an intelligence arm of the Department of Defense joined the challenge. In a document called "Note N–506, *Hunger USA 1968—A Critical Review*," the Institute for Defense Analysis [Science and Technology Division] unleashed an all-out attack on the credibility of the report.

Institute staff member Dr. Herbert Pollack accused the writers of the *Hunger USA* Board report of ignorance about nutrition and challenged virtually every physician and scientist quoted in the report. Taking the position that the government food programs work well, Dr. Pollack indicated that ignorance was at the root of any hunger and malnutrition problems in America.

Dr. Pollack's critique, so gratifying to the agriculture committees of Congress, stunned nutrition scientists at the country's leading universities. At Harvard, professor of nutrition Jean Mayer * said the Pollack document "was so riddled with enormous errors, so wrong in scientific, medical, and human terms as to be of a standard unacceptable for a first year graduate school." As Dr. Mayer and other doctors attacked the scientific validity of the Institute for Defense Analysis report, they also questioned Dr. Pollack's motives in preparing this venal, stinging polemic against a citizen effort to help poor and hungry Americans. (According to a Johnson Administration official, Pollack had been recruited by an Agriculture Department administrator, in the hope of destroying the credibility of the Board's criticism of Department of Agriculture food programs.) Dr. Mayer, concluding his review of the Pollack paper, said:

"Dr. Pollack, we all agree with you that because people forage in the dump for food does not prove scientifically that they are malnourished. It may mean that they, too, are ignorant. But let us at least agree that they, and many of our fellow citizens, have nutritional problems, and for God's sake, let us try to do something to help them. At the very least, don't snipe at those who want to help!"

As the investigators and counter-investigators locked

* Special Consultant on Nutrition to the President of the United States in 1969.

horns over the extent of hunger in America, a central question emerged—one which kept the argument alive in Washington and further postponed any emergency food aid. The question was legitimate: To what extent *does* lack of education account for severe malnutrition?

Most middle-class Americans—especially white Americans—quickly jumped to the conclusion that the poor suffer such gross ignorance about buying and eating nutritious food that no amount of food aid could improve their diets. "The poor spend all their money on coke and potato chips" was a common charge; another, that they throw away the free surplus commodities or trade them for beer. In Washington, liberal politicians generally blamed hunger on lack of money while conservatives dismissed malnutrition as a problem exclusively of ignorance. (This same pattern continued on into 1969, when President Nixon's most conservative advisers told him ignorance, rather than money, was the problem.)

The nutritionists who joined the parade of witnesses before the congressional investigators all agreed that shortages of *both* money and education contribute to the problems of the hungry poor. However, they did not credit poor people with any exclusive hold on nutritional ignorance. "We are a nation of nutritional illiterates," one professor said. "Yet we expect the poor to exercise some special discipline of nutrition knowledge that the rest of the country lacks."

Suggestions that the poor cannot live on a welfare or food stamp budget brought angry protests from those well-disciplined members of the middle class who have learned to spend their dollars proudly and frugally. After Chicago *Sun-Times* feature writer Anthony Monahan and his family of four lived on a welfare food allotment of $24.35 for one week, he wrote: "On the third day the oranges and apples ran out, on the fifth day, the potatoes, bacon, cereal, soup, and most of the vegetables were gone —but not forgotten."

The newspaper received a flood of protesting letters, although if the Monahan family had been one of the poorest in Chicago receiving food stamps, they would have had only $15 worth of groceries for the week. "A person who canot budget his money more wisely than Mr. Monahan does not deserve to be on welfare," one lady wrote.

The Chicago writer's experience was virtually echoed by an illiterate Negro housewife in DeKalb, Mississippi, who was asked whether her government food commodities lasted through the month. "Well, the meat don't," the mother of ten replied, and then continued slowly. "The cheese don't. The meal don't. The flour don't. The raisins don't. The peanut butter don't."

Her story brought an angry letter from a thrifty engineer in suburban Minneapolis, who described how his family of ten does not scrimp on $140 a month food allowance, or 15 cents per meal for each member of the family. "The Mississippians surely can grow gardens, gather their own wood free, and build better housing for themselves. . . . It is education—not food stamps and welfare—that the Mississippians need!"

If the engineer and his family of ten had been among the poorest buying food stamps, they would have had only $94 worth of groceries per month, rather than the $140 he successfully budgets. As a final test of his ingenuity the engineer might try feeding his family not on $140 montly but on $55 worth of surplus commodities, which is what this Negro family in DeKalb lives on.

The illiterate sharecropper undoubtedly could use some

help from the thrifty engineer on that one occasion at the end of the year when plantation owner Tom Stennis (a cousin of the senator) comes by to settle their accounts. Life for the sharecropper simply does not offer the opportunities for initiative that the Minnesotan and many middle-class Americans imagine. Mr. Stennis would not appreciate having his trees used for firewood or building material. Many plantation owners do not permit their valuable cotton land to be used for gardens. The sharecropper's children have little chance for a decent education in DeKalb—and even if the school were good, they often are too sick or lack the clothes to attend school. And finally, it is not a simple matter to pull up stakes and seek opportunity elsewhere. Even if he had the education and training to seek another job, the Stennis sharecropper said he would be afraid to leave if he owed Stennis any money—and he's not certain how his account now stands. (When Negro families flee the plantation, it is often at night to avoid that last accounting.)

Without disparaging the pride or the abilities of American families who skillfully economize and feed their families well on limited budgets, the few available studies on nutrition strongly indicate that being well-fed in America is largely a matter of dollars and *not* of nutritional knowledge. Evidence produced by the massive 1965 U.S. Department of Agriculture Food Consumption Survey strongly indicates that good nutrition is related directly to income—of families with less than $3,000 income, 36 percent had diets rated "poor," while in families with more than $10,000, only 9 percent of diets were rated "poor" (see chart, Appen. C.) The food consumption survey shows further that the amount of money spent for food was directly related to income, with families below $3,000 annual income averaging $17.00 per week for food, and families with more than $10,000 averaging $52.00. (See chart, Appen. C.)

Although the rise in income does parallel rise in education, the clinching argument that money is the prime determinant of dietary sufficiency for Americans is the 1965 Department of Agriculture study which shows the poor actually make *better* use of their nutritional dollars than do the well-to-do. The point is not that the poor are brighter nutritionally, but that they use less expensive foods in proportionately higher amounts and show enough judgment in choosing those foods to maximize their nutritional benefits. The family with under $3,000 income, for example, gets 3,150 calories of food energy per dollar while the family with more than $10,000 income buys only 2,100 calories with an average food dollar. (Again, the complete chart shows that those with progressively less income get more food value per dollar spent. See Appen. C.)

According to the food consumption study, the diets of the poor were most often lacking in calcium, Vitamin A value, and ascorbic acid—which are chiefly supplied by milk, milk products, vegetables, and fruits. These are the higher-priced items in a general diet, which poor people can least afford. Furthermore, every nutritional survey done by the Agriculture Department since the 1930s has shown that as income increases among the poor, these are precisely the products they buy more of.

In the heart of the nation's breadbasket, a 68-year-old Iowa widow who lives alone on $45.00 a month said, "I know I should be eating more meat to get the protein and most of the time I get a little hamburger almost every day. Doctor says I should be drinking fruit juices too, but

I figure I can get some Vitamin C from lemonade, it's a lot cheaper. . . . When you keep busy you don't mind being hungry so much."

A detailed study made among the poor residents of Cleveland, Ohio, proved that income and food purchasing power were the sole determinants in quality of diets. Even though comparisons were drawn as to race, educational level, etc., money still was the determining factor in improving diets. Asked what foods they would buy with more money, the poor again and again specified milk, meat, and fruit.

As the Agriculture Department battled to defend its food and farm programs in the late 1960's the food consumption surveys never were mentioned. If the Department of Agriculture had dared to dispute the belief in the laziness and ignorance of poor Americans by proving statistically that the poor used their food dollars more wisely than the well-to-do, no doubt it would only have succeeded in launching Chairmen Whitten and Poage on an investigation of the department itself.

"The poor spend money on non-essentials," say many righteous middle-class Americans. They complain about the buying of a car that can mean a poor man's only transportation to an occasional job, or a television set that is his only contact with *their* America. The poor man who buys a television set on "time" instead of saving for a food crisis may be hungry for more than just bread. For his children, television can be the one chance to enter vicariously a world that the rural black, for example, has never gained from a hundred years of segregated, inadequate schools. For the black man and his family, television opens up that strange soap-opera-situation-comedy society that is middle-class America. Above all it provides a new power—an end to isolation and a beginning of self-confidence as he sees others in his situation who are "doing something" about it.

Deep beneath the debate about whether malnutrition is a problem of money or education is a basic disagreement about the nature of life in this country, a basic difference of vision about what life really is like for the poor, about the nature of our social responsibility, and about what it takes for a poor man to "make it" in America. It is difficult to tell, at times, whether our different opinions come out of our various life experiences, or whether each of us has devised a view of life which is most convenient, most rewarding, and most reassuring.

These basic differences in outlook were spelled out in a confrontation between a congressman and a physician, both of whom have gone a long way toward their individual lifetime goals. The witness, Dr. Donald Gatch of South Carolina, and the questioner, Representative William Scherle of Iowa, contrast in appearance and in viewpoint. Dr. Gatch, slight, freckled, with an unruly thatch of brown hair, was born on the great plains of Nebraska and grew up on a ranch. He went southeast to practice medicine among the black poor of South Carolina, and made his mark there as an outspoken rebel physician, challenging the medical establishment of the nation to open its eyes to the wretched poor and to help them.

Representative Scherle, a towering man with close-cropped crew cut, a healthy suntanned face, and the hard muscles of a man who has done physical labor, was born in poverty in upstate New York, but went west and married a wealthy farmer's daughter in Iowa. He manages farms for himself and his father-in-law, assisted by generous government subsidy payments, and has made his mark in politics as an arch-conservative opposed to welfare programs.

As the two men met, Dr. Gatch was trying to explain to the House Education and Labor Committee * that the black poor of the South Carolina coastal areas were dying of hunger and medical neglect. Congressman Scherle questioned him:

"Why is it that poverty exists? . . . Why don't the people themselves, if you know the situation exists, help these [poor] people? You have welfare programs, you have a lot of social programs, you have leaders in the community."

Gatch: "First of all, they are unaware."

Scherle: "Couldn't you make them aware of it?"

Gatch: "I have tried. It is very difficult for a community to accept the fact that people are dying and are hungry, and live with it, without doing something about it, and so far, most of the South just denies that it exists."

Scherle: "But they know that it does."

Gatch: "Not actually. It is a funny thing what the automobile has done. It takes you past these houses. It doesn't take you in them. And it takes you past these people. . . ."

Scherle: "Are you telling me that this community completely closes their eyes to the situation and have become so hardened that they don't care?"

As Dr. Gatch tried to explain the phenomenon of affluent people who cannot see the dire poverty in their midst, the congressman angrily denied the existence of such blindness in America—especially in his district. Yet rural Mills County, Iowa, home of the strapping congressman, has a relatively high infant mortality rate, one of the

* The House Education and Labor Committee held hunger hearings in June 1968.

125

vague indices by which hunger and malnutrition are measured. Several hundred persons in Mills County rushed to buy food stamps when reluctant county officials finally consented to accept the federal program.

The question, then, does boil down to ignorance. But is it ignorance of the poor as to proper nutrition, or ignorance of most Americans as to the problems of the poor?

William H. Burson, Director of Family and Children Services for the State of Georgia, and a white southerner who believes there has been an effort to starve out the Negro, delivered his own sermon on the politics of ignorance as he characterized those who denied food to the poor in his state: "They are the sheriff who declares that anyone who goes to bed hungry is 'just sorry as hell' [no good]. They are the county commissioner who maintains his county cannot afford a food program even though he knows you know the county is solvent and has money in the bank. They are the farmer or contractor looking for cheap labor who insists, 'if you feed them, they won't work.' They are the Sunday school teacher who piously quotes from the Scriptures that 'the poor always ye have with you.' They are the prophet of doom who predicts that those given surplus commodities will 'feed them to the hogs' and those allowed to buy food stamps will swap them for beer and cigarettes. They are the well-fed businessman or banker who refuses to believe anyone is hungry because he never has been nor has he ever known anyone who has. They are the greedy merchant who charges he will be forced into bankruptcy if poor people are given food."

These people, Burson charged, are the ignorant.

# CHAPTER VIII

# Hunger and the Marketplace

JUST BEFORE CHRISTMAS IN 1967, JONATHAN W.
Sloat, Washington counsel for the Grocery Manufacturers of America, began receiving telephone calls from anxious executives in the food industry. Food manufacturers in New York, Chicago, St. Louis, and Minneapolis were perplexed, angry, and curious about a letter they had just received from Richard Boone of the Citizens' Board of Inquiry into Hunger and Malnutrition.

"I've never seen a letter quite so naïve—and one that caused so much controversy," an official of General Foods later confided. "Our response must have been rewritten 15 times, and there was quite a discussion about who should sign it."

Boone's letter revealed the basic facts about hunger and malnutrition in the United States and noted the inadequacy of government food aid programs in solving these urgent problems. Furthermore, the action-oriented Boone pointedly asked the chief executives of the industry—presidents of the major cereal, meat, dairy, and canned food companies—whether they and the government should be doing more to help the poor gain an adequate diet.

"Is the private sector devoting any special attention to the food needs of the chronically hungry poor?" he asked. "Why could low-cost fortified nutrients not be supplied to areas where the prevalence of malnutrition seems high? Should special attention be given to the problems of expectant mothers, newly-weaned infants, and to the aged poor? Are government food programs adequate—programs that reach only five million of 29 million poor?"

And finally, he asked the leaders of an industry that spends two billion dollars annually to advertise its products: "Can America gain freedom from hunger? If so, how?"

GMA lobbyist Sloat, a youthful lawyer in his mid-thirties, fended off industry questioners as best he could, while he tried to figure out just what the Citizens' Board of Inquiry was. Operating from his rather Spartan offices on K Street (the GMA's plush New York office, in contrast, is a showcase for the Association's members, with an entire red-carpeted corridor lined with full page, color ads of their products) just three blocks from the White House, Sloat has done his best to maneuver legislation favorable to profits for the $100 billion industry he represents—the nation's biggest business.

The provocative Boone letter had been sent to 75 of Sloat's member companies, and names of the 35 who bothered to reply sounded like a well-stocked grocery basket or a roster of the *Ladies' Home Journal* advertising pages. An evaluation of the 35 responses made several facts painfully clear:

- America's major food manufacturers professed to know little about the food problems of the poor.
- They felt that the answer to the needs of the hungry poor is mainly one of education and employment.
- They believed these problems, for which the food industry had no special public responsibility, were a matter for government attention.

Although a number of firms reported that they were working on fortified foods for undeveloped countries, they evidently could see no analogy between hunger in Afghanistan and hunger in Harlem. And some suggested that nothing can be done about problems of hunger in America because we don't know enough about it.

"I have difficulty seeing why major food manufacturers should be singled out to comment on problems of hunger and malnutrition," wrote W. Gardner Barker, President of Thomas J. Lipton, Inc., a major producer of soups, in addition to the famous tea ". . . The matter of hunger is, of course, related to economic well-being, and I fail to see why you should attribute any special competency to the food manufacturers to comment on economic well-being. . . ."

The economic well-being of the American food industry, however, has become a legendary success story of advanced technological and marketing developments. The American supermarket, an institution so unique that foreign visitors often want to visit one before seeing the historic sites, presents the affluent homemaker with such an overwhelming number of choices and conveniences that overeating and overweight have become a national concern. In spite of this overabundance on the grocery shelves, and unequaled profits in the history of the industry, most of the executives quizzed by the Board of Inquiry felt that the food industry had neither the know-how nor the obligation to deal with the unprofitable problems of feeding the hungry or to provide especially nutritious foods at low cost to help the poor. The poor were simply not part of the market for which cereal manufacturers competed with gimmick names and prizes in every box.

To scientists working in the field, however, the industry bears a special responsibility, because only it can apply available technical knowledge to feed the malnourished poor. One such scientist is Dr. Aaron Altschul, Special Assistant for Nutrition Improvement at the Department of Agriculture, an authority on the production and utilization of low-cost protein and vitamin fortified foods. In 1968, Dr. Altschul told the House Education and Labor Committee: "There is no excuse for not eliminating emergency problems of hunger and malnutrition in the United States within the next one to two years. Unless we are really stupid, the forces should now be in motion to knock out this problem!" [But a year later, neither government nor industry had moved.]

The 54-year-old Altschul, a lean, energetic extrovert, does not fit any of the stereotypes of ivory-tower, laboratory-bound scientists. He is equally at home discussing protein chemistry (he was a pioneer in the field) negotiating his way through the government bureaucracy, or discussing marketing economics with the captains of the food industry. His present goal is to convince the food industry to consider the needs of the poor in evaluating the markets for its products. During the past three years, Altschul has coaxed manufacturers into cooperating with the foreign aid program to develop fortified foods to combat hunger problems in underdeveloped countries. His results, along with the work of others, have been remarkable.

For example, in Guatemala and Colombia, the Quaker Oats Company is selling a protein-rich product called "Incaperina," a floury vegetable mixture made of corn, soy meal, and cottonseed meal, which is supplying adequate nutrition to poor Latin Americans at one-tenth the cost of powdered milk, one-fifth the cost of fresh milk, and one-third the cost of eggs. In El Salvador, the Pillsbury Company is selling a fortified powdered beverage mix, "Fresca Vida" (Fresh Life); Monsanto has an investment in the Hong Kong soft drink market with a fortified and tasty beverage called "Vitasoy"; the giant Coca Cola Corporation is test-marketing "Saci," a chocolate-flavored beverage in Brazil; and an Indian government-owned firm cannot keep up with the demand for "Modern," a protein-fortified bread which is so successful that black market operators are selling it slice by slice while competitors are trying to catch up by fortifying their bread products.

Swift and Company, the giant meat corporation, is working on a soybean-textured food for Brazil; International Milling Company is developing a high-protein wheat food for Tunisia; Dorr-Oliver is making a cottonseed protein product for use in India; and a South African firm is marketing protein-enriched drinks, candy, and other foods under the trade name "Pronutro."

In each case, modern technology in the food industry has supplied from oil seeds and test tubes the protein and vitamins most often missing from the diets of the malnourished and hungry poor. The American food industry also manufactured, for the U.S. Agriculture Department, CSM, a product made from corn, soy, and dried milk which supplies all the necessary nutrients and 70 percent of minimum calorie intake for children. Poverty children throughout the world, but not in the United States, received half a million pounds of this miraculous product from us in 1967—at a cost of two cents per day per child.

"We can now take children anywhere in the world and care for them nutritionally with the supplements that are now available," Dr. Altschul emphasized in testimony before the House Education and Labor Committee. He was there, this time, to urge development of such products as CSM to aid the poor in rural Mississippi, Appalachia, and the urban ghettoes of America. He ticked off the possibilities for nutritious and appetizing soft drinks; for candy bars containing 10 percent protein; for meat-like products made from soy beans; and for already-tested bread and cereals which can supply synthetic protein at a cost *per year* of 28 cents per child.

The eminent biochemist enthusiastically drove home this point: That American agriculture, industry, and government easily possess the technical ability to eliminate hunger and malnutrition in the United States now—merely by producing the same low-cost fortified foods used in the government's foreign-aid program. Dr. Altschul declared: "This goal can be reached by private industry—with not more than $50 million in government aid!" Altschul's dream has been blocked in part by other Agriculture Department officials who have discouraged development and use of synthetic or fortified foods which might represent competition for the department's farmer clients.

Private industry generally has not reacted to the challenge. It says that hunger in the United States is either a government problem, an economic problem, or no problem at all. The Borden Company's executive vice-president, for example, insists that his company's associates "are of the opinion that clinical malnutrition is not a public health problem in any sector of the United States." In answering the Citizens' Board of Inquiry questionnaire, this spokesman for the nation's biggest milk manufacturer sidestepped the question of whether government food programs, which reach only 20 percent of the poor, were adequate. The question "enters into broad areas of economics and political activity, and I therefore feel it would be impossible for me to comment."

Only the very naïve, however, could take this statement at face value, with its implication that food manufacturers and producers do not get involved "in economics and political activity." They have often involved themselves in issues with a direct impact on malnutrition among the poor. In fact, while its executives say "we are not concerned," the food industry's lobby, the GMA, worked actively to battle *against* legislation which might help feed the nation's hungry or protect consumers—rich and poor alike. The milk industry itself entered into a specific area of economic and political activity when it lobbied against government approval of a high-protein fish concentrate it felt would be a competitor.

Once a month, in the exclusive University Club in downtown Washington, the "Public Affairs Committee," lobbyists for GMA member companies, meet to talk about legislation of interest to the food industry. Jonathan Sloat takes part in these meetings, which are directed by his boss, GMA President George Koch (pronounced Cook).

Koch, a powerful, hardhitting professional Washington lobbyist (formerly chief lobbyist for Sears, Roebuck & Company) is well known on Capitol Hill. One of his associates describes him as having a "comprehensive attitude of opposition to just about everything in the way of social welfare legislation." Truth-in-packaging and other consumer legislation are also on his blacklist. The climate of Koch's monthly legislative sessions in the dark-paneled, rich-leather clubroom is described as negative—with law-blockage rather than law-making usually the objective. As one insider confided, "The attitude is one of complete opposition. We go over a list of all the bills. Then we get a position report on the status of each bill. If a bill has no chance of passing, we move on to the next item. If a bill has a chance of passing, it becomes a question of who can get to somebody [congressman or senator]. There's seldom any discussion about whether we *should* or *should not* oppose legislation."

The hunger issue came up at one of the 1968 sessions, and member Bryce Harlow, then lobbyist for Procter and Gamble * and now Assistant to President Nixon for congressional relations, questioned: "If we participate, won't government try to throw the entire hunger issue to the food industry?" This common attitude that the industry should "avoid involvement," might appear somewhat contradictory to another food industry shibboleth—that free enterprise should be able to solve problems without government interference.

Thus on the one hand, the industry wants to avoid involvement, leaving the matter to government; on the other hand, it is loath to let the government function without industry interference. The potent dairy lobby, for example, inspired a government restriction that until 1968 prohibited adding Vitamin A and D to nonfat dried milk which is shipped to the poor in 80 underdeveloped

---

* In the traditional Washington game of musical chairs in the "influence business," Harlow has been replaced at Procter and Gamble by Mike Manatos, a key White House congressional relations aide during the Kennedy and Johnson administrations.

countries and in some parts of the United States under the commodity programs. The giant dairy industry feared that the government-supplied milk might compete with whole milk in the marketplace. For the poor pregnant mother and her infant, however, this dried milk may represent the only hope for an adequate diet.

The food industry in 1967 played a significant role in temporarily killing legislation to supply emergency hunger aid. Although the grocery manufacturers' association now has "forgotten" it, GMA lobbyists quietly maneuvered against a bill to provide $50 million for two years for emergency food and medical aid to desperately malnourished Americans who are untouched by the food stamp or commodity distribution programs. The bill, however, was finally adopted, only after skillful advocates attached it to the antipoverty bill.

Soon after the dispute over emergency food aid, hunger lobbyist Robert Choate met GMA lobbyist Jonathan Sloat for the first time. "Oh, you represent the organization that lobbies against hungry people," sniped Choate in his most brittle Boston accent. Sloat mumbled that the legislation wasn't very good, then refused to discuss the matter.

Later, relations between the two men became more cordial, and when the GMA held its 1968 convention at the plush Greenbrier, a resort hotel in White Sulphur Springs, West Virginia, Choate implored Sloat to show the CBS documentary, "Hunger in America." (At that time, the Reverend Ralph David Abernathy was leading the poor People's Campaign in demonstrations at the U.S. Department of Agriculture, asking for better government food programs.) Hearing that the convention agenda was already too full, Choate asked whether the film might at

135

least be shown to wives accompanying their husbands to the convention. Sloat finally agreed to show the film—if inclement weather curtailed outdoor activities.

"Did you show the film?" Choate anxiously asked after Sloat returned from the Greenbrier.

"No," Sloat replied. "It never rained."

Hunger lobbyists were not able to invade the GMA convention, but less than a month later, GMA lobbyists made elaborate plans of their own to invade a couple of conventions. Grocery Manufacturers President Koch sought out well-placed GMA lobbyists to find out what plans were in store for "consumerism" and hunger issues in the two national political platforms for the upcoming party conventions. The industry, which believed malnutrition was strictly a government concern, jumped into the 1968 national political conventions, attempting to shape the scope of that government concern.

Since the GMA feared that a strong consumer or hunger plank would bind the nominee to "tough" programs, a Nabisco Company executive volunteered to lead a GMA probe to find out each Republican candidate's proposals on these issues and to influence members of the platform committee. And on the other side of the political fence, the GMA suite at the Sherman House was a flurry of activity during the Democratic Convention in Chicago. With tear gas and rioting in the streets, GMA lobbyists were concerned with downgrading consumer and hunger efforts for the campaign.

Robert Choate, disillusioned by finding so few good corporate citizens, laid out the industry's view in a stinging 1968 memo to the Citizens' Board of Inquiry:

"We cannot find one single instance of a major food manufacturer supporting a piece of poverty welfare legislation bringing adequate food to the poor unless that legislation meant increased sales for that food line. In their desire to keep the 'market open' even at the poverty end of the population and in their desire to avoid 'government intervention' they have supported . . . denial of government-subsidized food to the hungry residents of the United States."

In the same memo, Choate, a wealthy Republican who probably knows more about the domestic hunger issue than any other businessman in America, had also noted, "We have spoken with many [food company leaders] who cannot admit that there may be those in the United States who cannot afford food; many have gross misconceptions of the coverage of the present-day government programs. These same executives frequently claim that education of the poor is the answer. *We believe education of the poor to use nonavailable foodstuffs to be an escapist phrase.*"

After a year spent in fruitless effort to enlist meaningful support from the food industry, Choate found the food aid reformers and the traditionally conservative industry to be poles apart in their conceptions of what is at stake. The food manufacturers have often answered such challenges as Boone's and Choate's by pointing to the steadily declining percentage of American income spent for food. Indeed, many food executives seem to believe that they already have made their contribution to the hungry poor through the collective genius of the American food industry. As Dale W. McMillen, Jr., President of the Central Soya Company, wrote to the Citizens' Board of Inquiry: "The U.S. food industry is one of the great success stories in history. Today, the U.S. consumer is spending less than 18 percent of his income to be the best-fed consumer in the history of the world. . . . The new food technology has made low-cost and nutritious foods available to the hungry poor. Their acquisition and use of such foods is a problem which is essentially an economic and educational one."

This food executive, as well as Secretaries of Agriculture, all succumbed to a statistic that contributes absolutely nothing to solving the problems of the hungry poor. In fact, the much heralded 17.6 percent figure that Americans supposedly spend for food is a misleading statistic.

The National Commission on Food Marketing, in its exhaustive 1965 study, concluded that the "declining share of consumer income spent for food is not evidence of superior performance by the food industry." The commission noted that the percentage of income spent for food has dropped mostly because the middle class is already well fed and so does not buy more food when income rises, and because farm commodity prices have not risen in 20 years. In addition, the commission noted that families in low-income areas have gained the least from modern food distribution geared to mass markets; prices are usually higher in the smaller independent stores most common in low-income neighborhoods. Thus, while the rich are spending less, the poor actually spend more of their income for food. The fact that "Americans" spend 17.6 percent of income for food means little to those countless American families with $500 to $3,500 annual income and a number of mouths to feed, who must spend at least 30 to 100 percent of their meager funds to have any chance for an adequate diet.

As hunger investigators delved further into the issue of food manufacturing, far more serious questions arose concerning the industry's contributions to the nutrition of Americans, both rich and poor. Consumer advocate Ralph Nader pointed out to Congress that the food industry

138

spent only $12 million on basic food research, while in the same year it spent $1.3 billion on advertising. In numerous products, the evidence is mounting that less nutrition is being provided today, as the supermarket shelves are filled with more glamorous packaging, processing, and advertising.

Dr. Jean Mayer, eminent nutritionist at Harvard, has severely criticized the baby food industry for changing the composition of its product strictly from a profit motive and at the cost of less nutrition for infants. He noted a steady increase in the amount of starches and sugar added to baby food meats, fruits, and vegetables. The starch and sugar cost less and provide fewer essential nutrients in the meal, he explained.

The Senate Select Committee on Nutrition explored the nutrition of baby food in 1969 hearings at which scientists questioned the safety of adding salt and monosodium glutimate (MSG) to baby foods. These ingredients are added strictly to appeal to the mother's taste. After first declining to testify, executives of the H. J. Heinz Co. and Gerber Products Co., the leading sellers of baby foods, finally appeared to defend the safety of their products. The Heinz company, however, declined to bring along its own research chief, who for several years had been trying to persuade the company to remove MSG and to limit salt in its baby foods.

Dr. Thomas A. Anderson, chief of Heinz's Nutritional Research Laboratory, had urged development of a more nutritious baby food. Top company officials refused, however, fearing that Heinz might lose ground to Gerber in undertaking a task as tricky as "selling nutrition." At first, Heinz officials denied to the senate committee that Dr. Anderson had recommended changing the formula. Later, confronted with copies of Anderson's letters to a doctor, the executives shifted their story. Anderson never had made his recommendations "to the company," explained Heinz executive I. J. Hutchings, but only to his immediate superior.

Dr. Jean Mayer points out that modern processing and packaging methods in other foods often result in a loss of nutritional adequacy. The retention of Vitamin C content in orange juice has been increasingly endangered, he said, as processing methods changed from canned juice to frozen juice in tin cans and finally to juice in cardboard containers which may be too porous to retain Vitamin C adequately.

Dr. Arnold Schaefer, director of the Department of Health, Education, and Welfare's National Nutrition Survey, told a Senate committee that the food industry is acting irresponsibly with at least three basic products of vital nutritional importance. His points were:

• Much non-iodized salt is sold today despite the fact that doctors are discovering a recurrence of endemic goiter (caused by lack of iodine). Some manufacturers and grocers charge several cents more for iodized salt although the actual cost of adding iodine to salt is infinitesimal.

• Manufacturers of bread and flour products today are producing far more products without iron enrichment than they did 25 years ago, when virtually all flour was enriched because the Army required fortification for its massive food purchases.

• Milk manufacturers are selling more milk without Vitamin A and D fortification and are charging several cents more for enriched milk, although the cost of enrichment actually is only a few cents per hundreds of gallons.

Schaefer contends that in each of these cases adequate

nutrition has been sacrificed for the profit motive. The government, he argues, should require enrichment of all flour and Vitamin fortification of all milk—particularly since milk is the most suitable product for Vitamin D fortification. Non-iodized salt should be sold only as a special diet product, he adds.

Another congressional investigation has disclosed that the fat content of frankfurters and similar products has climbed steadily over the last 20 years and now averages more than 33 percent, while protein content has declined. Although meat manufacturers argue that they have increased fat content to suit consumers' taste preferences, nutritionists say the profit motive again has been the governing factor. The meat manufacturers also have strongly resisted a proposed regulation requiring them to list by percentage the amount of fat and protein content in their products. "We are now better informed about the nutritional content of the food we feed our dogs, cattle, and pigs than about human food," Representative Neal Smith of Iowa told Congress, as he noted that farmers demand to know the nutritional content of feeds for their animals.

Senator George McGovern of South Dakota began investigating the fat content of frankfurter-type products because of the heavy reliance by the poor on such cheaper meats. An advisory committee to the school lunch program recommended in 1969 that no more than 25 percent fat be permitted for hot dogs used in the school lunch program. The same committee of nutritionists expressed great concern in discovering that the caloric content of many school lunch program meals consisted of almost 40 percent fat. Nutritionists such as Dr. Mayer and government scientists like Dr. Altschul believe the school lunch program offers tremendous potential for improving nutrition of poor children through the use of fortified foods.

*141*

Yet the vested interests of agribusiness and of the school lunch administrators repeatedly have blocked improvements which could come from use of fortified products or from the services of skilled food caterers. The farm lobbyists are concerned about losing the school lunch program as an avenue for the disposal of several hundred million dollars annually in surplus commodities. The school lunch administrators are worried about losing their jobs to outside catering firms.

After several years of discussions with scientists employed by the nation's major food manufacturing firms, Dr. Altschul is convinced that "the technicians are chomping at the bit" to provide innovative, low-cost fortified foods for the poor. Sadly, the adventurous and innovative spirit of the researchers often has not been shared by the marketing people who dominate this industry. Two cases in point occurred in 1969.

In one instance, the director of research for a major national bakery developed a highly enriched bread which could supply important nutritional benefits to the poor at low cost. The company's marketing management turned down his product on the grounds that the margin of profit would be too low. In the other case, a scientist for a major baby food manufacturer proposed marketing a line of products with much higher nutrient content and less sugar and starches. He suggested an advertising campaign comparing the relative nutrient content of this product and those produced by rival firms. Top management dismissed the idea as one that might disrupt the industry at a time when profits already were at record highs.

Publicly, the grocery manufacturers almost always say that nutrition education, which would teach people how to use available foods, rather than more income for the poor or fortification of low-cost foods, is the answer to hunger and malnutrition. When questioned by the Citizens' Board of Inquiry in 1967, they referred the issue to the prestigious Nutrition Foundation, which they support with sizeable annual grants, and which, according to the president of the Lipton Company, "uses its resources in the interest of proper nutrition for the American public both through its research and its educational arms."

Even though the executives suspected that "there is a lot of money misspent on the Kool-Aid and potato chip meal" which could be better spent on dried milk, soups, fruit, and other items, the Nutrition Foundation was not much help in providing answers, asserting that this type of "education" was not within its realm of competence, and referring the Citizens' Board to nonexistent "studies by federal agencies and universities." The Nutrition Foundation declined to support the Board of Inquiry's hunger probe, leading hunger lobbyist Choate and others to wonder whether this foundation had any function besides puffing up the food industry.

Another potential source of industry involvement in feeding the poor was the Agribusiness Council, formed in 1967 to "stimulate and increase efforts of the American agribusiness community in alleviating the problems of the food supply in developing countries." Although a chief council topic is the development and distribution of fortified and synthetic foods, chairman Henry J. Heinz II, board chairman of the company which bears his name, showed no interest in expanding the Agribusiness Council's concern to include problems at home as well as those overseas.

Even though the American food industry as a whole has responded negatively to suggestions that it might become involved or assist in solving domestic hunger prob-

*143*

lems, a few food manufacturers have recognized the irony of using food industry technology abroad, but not at home, and have expressed interest in solving the problem with this technology.

Leaders of Pepsico, General Mills, and Pet, Inc., thought something should be done, and William F. Quinn, president of the Dole Co., offered broad encouragement and advice to the Board of Inquiry. The Quaker Oats Company reported on a successful pilot project it had initiated in the Chicago slums, with food preparation classes disguised as enjoyable nonwelfare projects for housewives with the very lowest income and education.

Since initial contacts were made in 1967, there is some slight evidence that the industry has begun to feel the moral sting on the hunger issue and to sense the danger of damage to its public image. GMA President Koch in exasperation "to get Choate off our backs," ordered TV spots on nutrition to be shown on educational channels and assigned a task force to study the issue and draw up a "position paper."

This GMA position paper on hunger and malnutrition, presented August 30, 1968, suggested actions which were at least a beginning. It urged that the GMA work with the government in school lunch and other child feeding programs; encourage local officials to participate in the food stamp program; work with federal agencies to develop solutions on a regional basis; encourage efforts to study the nutritional adequacy of regional and ethnic diets; and support public service nutrition education.

One imaginative suggestion was the idea of promoting a "fortified food fair"—since "the inventory of fortified foods in all forms in our research labs would stock a fairsized supermarket." The private GMA paper also departed from tradition by supporting the use of fish pro-

144

tein concentrate (a flourlike product made from whole fish) to fortify food.

Agribusiness generally has opposed development of low-cost nutrients, as possible marketplace competition, and supported Food and Drug Administration restrictions on sale of fortified foods. Such was the case with fish protein concentrate. Because of opposition from the competing milk and milling industries, the Food and Drug Administration has restricted its sale to one-pound containers, thereby limiting its commercial use. When challenged to provide more low-cost fortified foods, industry officials often have replied that they are held back by FDA regulations, but fail to mention that industry influence has played an important role in shaping the regulations.

Although a few food industry eyes have been opened to the possibilities of profit from low-cost nutrition, the debate on education versus fortification still continues. Here, too, the industry often takes contradictory public positions. For example, General Mills executive Arthur Odell told a Senate committee that education was the answer to nutrition problems among the poor, since the poor will not buy any product with the stigma of "poor man's protein."

Why can't low-cost, high-protein products be marketed to the general public, including the poor, Odell was asked by a reporter.

"You can't sell nutrition," he replied. "Hell, all people want is coke and potato chips."

In this fashion, the industry generally has urged education as the answer and then disclaimed any responsibility, or even ability, to help provide it.

Most advocates for the hungry poor readily acknowledge the importance of increased nutrition education, but

*145*

declare that income, rather than ignorance is at the root of the problem. Dr. Altschul, the nutritional biochemist who urges fortification, and fortification now, insists that "the poor are not any more ignorant about food nutrition than anyone else; they just have less money."

The hunger issue had developed sufficient political momentum by 1969 that the Grocery Manufacturers of America volunteered to meet with the government and to participate in a White House Conference on Food, Nutrition, and Health.

An incident during the planning of this conference illustrates the influence to which industry responds rapidly. Dr. Jean Mayer, director of the conference, noted that many new foods lack all of the essential nutrients of the products they replace. As an example, Dr. Mayer cited "Tang," which he said does not contain the potassium found in orange juice. A hypertension patient ordered to drink orange juice would be in trouble, Dr. Mayer said, if he relied on Tang since the orange juice is prescribed specifically for its potassium. Among those at the meeting with Mayer was Dr. Paul Pearson, director of the industry-sponsored Nutrition Foundation. Within three hours after the meeting, the president of General Foods called Mayer to tell him that the company would put potassium into Tang.

It remains to be seen whether the food industry will respond only when its image is threatened or whether it really will concentrate on giving the poor more nutrition for less money.

# CHAPTER IX

# The Politics of Hunger—Round Two

FOR THOSE WHO BELIEVED THAT HUNGER PRO-
vided a meaningful new metaphor for the issue of poverty
in affluent America, 1968 was a chaotic, unpredictable
year of surprising battles won, of bitterest defeat, and—
through the worst of it all—a glimmer of hope for the
future.

Round One in the fight to end hunger in America had
produced a winning legislative decision. Just days before the new year began, Representative Albert Quie's
amendment to the Economic Opportunity Act promised
to bring a few million dollars of emergency aid to the
hungry. Compared to the real need of several billion, the
victory was small, symbolic, and only a beginning. It
made little impact on Washington, because hunger was a
primary concern only to a handful of politicians, and the
President of the United States was not among them.

In his first message of 1968, President Johnson tried to buoy the confidence of a troubled nation. But despite his State of the Union optimism, the President faced a strong, disruptive current in the society. He was bedeviled by a war which grew more unpopular by the minute, by a poverty program that had naïvely overpromised and underperformed, by a black revolution, by an inflationary economy that might wipe out prosperity in one flash of economic heat, and by a war-burdened budget that simply would not be balanced—even with a tax increase. And to get the tax increase, an exasperated President concluded that he would have to submit to virtual blackmail from the most conservative members of the House of Representatives, men like Appropriations Committee Chairman George Mahon and Ways and Means Committee Chairman Wilbur Mills. For 36 years, men such as Mahon and Mills, from the small towns of the South and the Midwest, had fought every step of the way against initiatives to build federally implemented social responsibility into government. Although such men never ceased their battle, usually they had lost, and many of them were all but forgotten. But in 1968 they had a chance to score a tremendous victory against the welfare state. If Lyndon Johnson wanted a tax bill from them, they said, he would have to halt further increases in the War on Poverty, which, like the war in Vietnam, needed replenished supplies once it was raging. All the political risks would belong to the President. He would have to cut up his own programs, his proudest accomplishments. They would just sit on the tax bill, and wait.

As he prepared his budget and programs for 1968, Lyndon Johnson for the second consecutive year ignored a secret task force report pleading for urgent action against domestic hunger and malnutrition. When Joseph

Califano, Johnson's chief assistant for domestic affairs, brought him the report, the President quickly dismissed the idea of a new program—even one involving only the sparse $300 million recommended by the task force. The report failed to prove the existence of hunger and malnutrition, Johnson said; it showed him neither who was suffering nor where they lived. The report, based on estimates, lacked definite, "hard" numbers, and he was not convinced that hunger in America was a serious problem or that an emergency existed.

The President may well have reasoned that a big food program would be one more irritant to the congressional conservatives who held power over his tax bill—Mills of Arkansas, Mahon of Texas, and their Agriculture confederates Jamie Whitten, Bob Poage, Allen Ellender, and Spessard Holland.

President Johnson's State of the Union foreboding about a new spirit abroad, a "restlessness, a questioning," quickly proved accurate as Minnesota Senator Eugene McCarthy, on a wave of anti-Vietnam votes, came close to defeating him in the New Hampshire Presidential primary. Within a few days after New Hampshire, Robert Kennedy's own restlessness brought the New York Senator out to challenge the President, and as the Wisconsin primary drew near, all of the polls that Lyndon Johnson carried in his pocket told him McCarthy might well defeat him there.

The politics of hunger and the politics of Vietnam were contrasted on March 31 in two powerful, surprising speeches, one far overshadowing the other. President Lyndon B. Johnson and Dr. Martin Luther King, Jr., both spoke to the nation on that Sunday.

From the pulpit of the vast Washington Cathedral, Dr. King told an attentive congregation why he planned to bring 3,000 poor people to Washington for a live-in demonstration. Struggling to maintain the civil rights movement as a nonviolent protest, King was determined to expose the plight of poverty by having the poor show how they lived and tell Congress and the nation in their own words what poverty was all about. He would dramatize the problems of poverty as his civil rights movement in the South had dramatized racial injustice. King and his Southern Christian Leadership Conference were in contact with the food aid reformers, and the issue of hunger and malnutrition was certain to be a focal point for the demonstration.

"It is morally wrong for a nation to spend $50,000 to kill a Viet Cong soldier and just $53 a year to help a poor person in the United States," King told his well-dressed white audience.

That same night, President Johnson announced to the nation he would not seek reelection. In his remaining ten months in office, he would attempt to find peace in Vietnam. For three days, the newly liberated President made progress with the tax bill and the war as North Vietnam agreed to peace talks.

Then, on April 4, the roof caved in on any Presidential plans to move forward with domestic legislation and find domestic peace. Dr. King was murdered by a sniper as he stood on a motel balcony in Memphis, and within hours riots swept the ghettoes of American cities.

Jarred by terror, and by four days of rioting which left a two-mile corridor of rubble, race-conscious Washington nervously awaited the poor people who headed toward the capital to fulfill Dr. King's last dream.

Despite the demoralizing effects of yet another political assassination and an increasingly reactionary mood in Congress and the nation, the food aid reformers still

150

hoped that the demonstration would provide human appeal and a sense of decency which would compel the President, Congress, and the nation to provide aid for the hungry poor. The efforts of more than a year's work had built to a climax and the scene was still set, they hoped, for a major breakthrough on the food issue in 1968.

Within one week in mid-April:

The Citizen's Board of Inquiry issued its report citing widespread hunger and malnutrition; the Committee on School Lunch Participation * (also funded by the bold Field Foundation) issued "Their Daily Bread," a study documenting the failure of the National School Lunch Program to help the poor child; Senator George McGovern and 38 other senators called for creation of a Senate Select Committee to study hunger and malnutrition; a bipartisan House group prepared to take similar action; and the Senate by an overwhelming vote rolled over the objections of Senator Allen Ellender's Agriculture Committee and authorized a $96 million pilot program to feed preschool children living in poverty, and CBS readied its hour-long television special on hunger. The timing of all these events was not entirely coincidental.

The Citizens' Board of Inquiry and the school lunch committee (ably led by Jean Fairfax of the Legal Defense Fund) prepared release of their studies for maximum public impact, which hopefully would stimulate action in Congress and the White House. Working behind the scenes toward that end, Kennedy legislative aide Peter Edelman, Poverty Subcommittee Counsel Bill Smith, Mc-

---

* The committee was sponsored by five women's organizations: United Church Women, National Board of the Y.W.C.A., National Council of Catholic Women, National Council of Jewish Women, National Council of Negro Women.

Govern aide Benton Stong, and hunger lobbyist Robert Choate planned daily strategy for steering hunger legislation past hostile Senate and House Agriculture Committees. The role of these men became doubly important because Kennedy and Clark both were now out campaigning—Kennedy for the Presidency, Clark for re-election—and were away from the daily Washington legislative struggle. As a start, the strategists helped stimulate a new set of legislative leaders and suggested to them a plan of action.

Meaningful action in the Senate, they decided, could best be achieved by creating a brand new Select Committee with the freedom to explore the politics of hunger wherever they led. This would include, obviously, a critical probe of the entire agriculture power structure.

The Senate does not take lightly to forming new committees, especially committees that might challenge established institutions. The proposed hunger committee, therefore, would require a skillful congressional genesis—because conservative members of the Agriculture Committee were certain to regard the creation of a new nutrition group as a move to strip their control over food aid programs. In an artful display of political astuteness, the food aid reformers decided that members of the Agriculture Committee itself should lead the fight.

Ellender and other southern powers watched in dismay as a bipartisan group from their own committee—Democrats George McGovern and Walter Mondale, Republicans Mark Hatfield and Caleb Boggs—toured the Senate signing up additional sponsors for their resolution. With four of his own members advocating the new group, Ellender could hardly complain that their purpose was to bypass the Agriculture Committee. The resolution was carefully worded so that it would escape the jurisdiction of the Agriculture Committee and the equally conservative Rules Committee. McGovern aide Ben Stong, a legislative veteran, designed the proposal so that Joseph Clark's friendly Poverty Subcommittee would officially consider it. In the process, he taught Choate and the other food aid reformers how to use traditional political maneuvering to win new objectives.

The day after the Citizens' Board of Inquiry report was issued, McGovern took the Senate floor with a copy of *Hunger, USA* in his hand. He introduced his resolution, now sponsored by 38 other senators, to form the Senate Select Committee on Nutrition and Human Needs, and to investigate issues raised in *Hunger, USA*. The Senate soon approved the new committee.

In the House of Representatives, the food aid reformers planned their strategy to steer meaningful legislation around the jurisdiction of Bob Poage and his ultra-conservative House Agriculture Committee. The ideal solution would be for the more liberal Education and Labor Committee to invade Poage's territory. The key to this maneuver was held by House Education and Labor Chairman Carl Perkins of Kentucky, a moderate Democrat who respected House and party customs, and thus would be unlikely to challenge fellow chairman Poage. But Bob Choate devised a plan to win over Perkins. Democratic Representative Thomas Foley and Republican Charles Goodell rounded up most of the members of Perkins' own committee, plus several from Poage's committee, to request that hunger hearings be held by Education and Labor. Perkins, facing political embarrassment, could no longer resist. When Foley and Goodell staged a press conference of their *ad hoc* coalition to urge action on the hunger issue, Perkins agreed to hold hearings. Seated in the front row as a spectator at the press conference, Agriculture Chairman Poage sputtered angrily about usurping congressional powers and holding needless hearings.

If the Poor People's Campaign would have a positive impact on Congress and on the public, and if President Lyndon Johnson would cooperate, there was now enough groundwork for legislative action.

When Dr. King planned the Poor People's Campaign, he stated its objectives only in the broadest terms—massive new programs for jobs and housing, and a guaranteed annual income. When his successor as head of the Southern Christian Leadership Conference, the Reverend Ralph David Abernathy, arrived in Washington on April 28 with an advance delegation of 100 poor people, he had few specific objectives in mind. On this preliminary visit, Abernathy, planned only "to present the leadership of this country with a moral manifesto that talks in terms of needs"—needs for jobs, housing, income, land, food, and self-determination. In his view, details of the program would follow naturally, suggested by the dynamics of the protest movement as it developed. This had been the pattern of several of Dr. King's successful campaigns in the South.

A number of campaign aides, however, tried to convince Abnernathy that he must be considerably more specific when he began to visit various government departments the next morning. Washington simply does not react, they said, to broad moral manifestoes. If the poor people were to function effectively as Washington lobbyists, they must have definite programs for both legislative and executive action. For specifics, Abernathy then turned to Marian Wright, who had inspired Kennedy and Clark in Mississippi a year earlier and who now served as the Poor People's Campaign chief liaison officer with the government. Assisted by Kennedy aide Peter Edelman, Poverty Subcommittee Counsel Bill Smith, and black officials in the Johnson Administration, Miss Wright drew up a practical program to fulfill the high promise of new social legislation. Aside from a call for major new housing and job programs, the emphasis was on reform of existing programs and institutions. It was a radical program, but only in the sense that it called on cynical Washington to practice fully the spirit and intent of laws already on the books.

The Justice Department was asked to begin enforcing civil rights laws which had been passed in dramatic, filibuster-breaking debate, and then given only minimal enforcement attention. The Department of Health, Education, and Welfare was told to reform its welfare program rules, so that they provided elementary justice to welfare recipients. The Office of Economic Opportunity was asked to make "maximum feasible participation of the poor" in its programs a reality rather than a motto. When the Poor People's issues list turned to the Agriculture Department, Miss Wright applied her special knowledge and interest in food programs. The Poor People's Campaign demanded that the Agriculture Department carry out the reforms recommended the previous week by the Citizens' Board of Inquiry and the Committee on School Lunch Participation: free and reduced-price food stamps, more and better commodities, free lunches for the nation's poor children, emergency action in the Board of Inquiry's "256 hunger counties," and fulfillment of the Administration's 1967 pledge to place a food program in each of the nation's 1,000 poorest counties.

The next morning, April 29, 1968, with neatly typed proposals in hand, Reverend Abernathy launched the Poor People's Campaign in Washington.

As the 100-member delegation made its way about the capital, Washington's sedate business-suit-and-briefcase world raised its eyebrows. Perhaps official Washington was startled because it had expected to greet another well-organized delegation of businessmen, farmers, or doctors —each delegate wearing a neat identification tag and conscientiously carrying out his assignment to knock at the door of his congressman. Instead the capital found itself confronted by a noisy, emotional group of people whose principal common bond was a shared experience of misery

Wherever it went, the group was disorganized and late. This in itself was enough to cause shock waves—who ever heard of poor supplicants keeping a busy Cabinet officer waiting for two hours? There was a tendency for everyone to talk at once, and there was confusion about where the next appointment would be. But there was also—if Washington could find the sensitivity to filter out the unaccustomed distractions—an intense, honest presentation of critical human issues which no $100,000-a-year corporate lobbyist-lawyer could have framed as effectively.

Mrs. Martha Grass, an American Indian from Ponca City, Oklahoma, broke into sobs before a Senate committee as she described the life of her people: "It is just a miracle we keep alive. Our men break their health pitching hay for two cents a bale because they can't even get dishwashing jobs. We shared this country with you, but you took all of it and we're starving. It's very hard when your child asks for something to eat and you've got nothing to give him when all around you see how rich everybody else is in this country."

Emotion poured from the lips of these poor people, who had been motivated strongly enough to come to Washington. In a packed conference room at the Agriculture

Department, Secretary Freeman and his top aides heard an angry black lady from Baltimore conclude her description of a day of poverty: "I go to sleep every night with rats for my pillow, roaches for my blanket."

As this group poured out of Freeman's conference room on April 30, 1968, the words of "We Shall Overcome" rang through the halls of the huge government building. Abernathy, singing and clasping two marchers by the hand, led the way. "They killed Martin Luther King but this poor people's campaign was his last dream," Abernathy preached in the Department lobby. "His spirit is here. We are going to prove to the assassin or assassins—you may kill his body but not his dream. We have come here today and will remain for days, weeks, and months if necessary to do away with an island of poverty—to build a bridge to the mainland. We are determined we are not going to beg for our rights any longer but will demand them. We have made up our minds and there will be no new business in this country until it takes care of the old business."

Abernathy met with both Republican and Democratic congressional leaders who affirmed his right to petition the Congress for redress of grievances. He assured them his demonstration would be peaceful. It was all very polite. And, as he left each Cabinet office, Abernathy spelled out the timetable for the campaign. The government would be given *ten days* to study the demands of the Poor People's Campaign. "At the end of that time," Abernathy said, "we will be back—not with 150 as today but 3,000 to 5,000 strong and we will demand answers. We are going to back up our words with the most militant, nonviolent direct action in this country's history."

As best he could, President Johnson was preparing for an extremely delicate task. While he bargained with arch-conservatives in Congress over billions of dollars in spending cuts as the price of a tax bill, he also was searching for positive responses to defuse the potentially incendiary Poor People's Campaign; thousands of poor people were pouring into Washington, less than three weeks after the worst of the King assassination riots.

From his White House office, Joe Califano dialed the Secretary of Agriculture. "The President wants you to work up two sets of responses to the Poor People's Campaign," Califano told Orville Freeman. "He wants a list of things we can do *without* congressional action, and another list of the responses which will require legislation. This whole thing is absolutely top secret. I want to emphasize that. We've got to maintain the highest security."

The plan was so secret that Califano, unwilling to risk memos that might be seen by many eyes, delivered the President's instructions verbally to each member of the Cabinet.

At an April 30 Cabinet meeting, the President emphasized the need for speed in developing answers to Abernathy. Careful timing was needed, the President said, in order to coordinate the intricate tax maneuverings in Congress with the effort to satisfy the poor people, so that solving one problem did not adversely affect the other. To expedite and coordinate the operation, Califano assigned a White House staff member to work with each department of government.

DeVier Pierson, a young Oklahoman, drew the Agriculture Department assignment. Moving swiftly, Pierson called a White House meeting on May 2 to discuss responses to Abernathy's demands for better food programs. At last, the Agriculture Department appeared eager for reform. Moreover, Pierson found an influential White House enthusiast in Presidential assistant Charles Murphy, a longtime friend of the President and an old hand Washingtonian whose career had included service both as Undersecretary of Agriculture and as a lawyer-lobbyist. He had the special experience to know that Abernathy's charges against the Agriculture Department were well founded.

"We've never had a commitment to eliminate hunger in this country and it's about time we had one," said Murphy to the group of Agriculture and Budget Bureau officials at the meeting. Then he passed around a copy of a food proposal he had given the President two days earlier.

"Despite all our efforts," Murphy wrote the President, "we have never comes to grips in a systematic, total way with the problem of hunger in America. . . . Despite the best efforts of the Agriculture Department, [its] programs do not come close to meeting the need."

Murphy's plan called for immediate spending of $170 million to improve the commodity and food stamp programs and to provide more free school meals for poor youngsters. Furthermore, he proposed a $2.5 billion program to guarantee "that by 1970 or 1971 every American will be given a reasonable opportunity to avoid hunger or malnutrition which affects him through no fault of his own." A $2 billion food stamp program would be operated like a negative income tax, with stamps to be distributed by the Internal Revenue Service. Stamps would cost less and the poor would receive more of them.

The Murphy proposal brought immediate and eager support from Agriculture Secretary Freeman, who for more than a year had taken the brunt of food program criticism.

At the next White House meeting on May 6, Agriculture Undersecretary John Schnittker was given two days to work up final details on a legislative package which, it was expected, the President then would deliver to legislative leaders. The proposal called for spending $100 million of Section 32 funds to add more nutritious foods to the commodity program, and also requested an additional $200 million from Congress to begin expansion and reform of the food stamp program.

As the massive march on Washington approached, enthusiastic officials at both the Agriculture Department and in those White House offices closest to the President expected a "go" signal from Lyndon Johnson at any moment. The green light never came on, and one reason was clearly stated when the President sent Charlie Murphy's proposal back to him.

"That's something to consider," the President said, "but *nothing* must be permitted to interrupt the negotiations with Congress to get that tax bill!" The President turned down the proposal on the grounds it would endanger his maneuvers to win the needed $10 billion of new revenue.

As the Agriculture Department and the White House staff hurriedly worked up food reform programs and pushed them toward the President's desk, Lyndon Johnson was undergoing the single most trying period of his year-long effort to pass the tax bill. At a secret White House meeting on April 30 (the same day he urged his Cabinet to plan responses for Abernathy), the President thought he had reached a compromise with Ways and Means Chairman Mills and Appropriations Chairman Mahon for a 10 percent surcharge tax increase, purchased from them with promises for a $4 billion spending cut in 1969, a $10 billion reduction in obligational authority, and an $8 billion reduction of spending authorized in earlier years but not yet spent. But within 48 hours Arkansas conservative Mills denied he had agreed to a deal. Angered by Mills in particular and Congress in general, the President publicly accused the Congress of virtual blackmail on the tax issue as he delivered an angry, 1,200-word off-the-cuff response at a press conference. By May 8, when he received the food aid proposal from Schnittker, the tax bill was back on track again with Mills, but problems were coming from a different direction. House and Senate conferees had approved the tax package provisional to a $6 billion spending cut. Liberals were infuriated and Johnson was worried that deep cuts in basic Great Society legislation would be required.

A food aid law might be desperately needed by the hungry poor, but Lyndon Johnson was concerned at that point only with the mentality of men who could defeat a tax bill—men like Congressman O. C. Fisher, of Texas, who said of the approaching Poor People's Campaign, "The invading hordes headed this way will leave crime, immorality, bloodshed, arson, and looting in their wake." The Poor People were being reviled daily on the House and Senate floors, the House Public Works Committee voted to keep the campaigners from camping on government property, and Senator John McClellan of Arkansas warned the White House about possible subversive motives.

Publicly, the President tried to maintain equilibrium and hold the middle ground. "We do expect the poor will be better served after that viewpoint is presented," he said, "though every person in the Capital should be aware of the possibilities of serious consequences, flowing from assemblage of large numbers over any protracted period of time in the seat of government where there is much work to be done and very little time to do it."

Although the poor people were just starting out from the Deep South, President Johnson already had assumed their stay in Washington would be a long one—for hunger was becoming a principal issue of the campaign, and the President silently had rejected plans to feed the hungry poor.

# CHAPTER X

# The Poor People and the War President

FROM THE DUST-PAVED STREETS OF "FROGTOWN" in Savannah, Georgia, to the narrow alleys of the unnamed black quarter in Demopolis, Alabama, young lieutenants of the Southern Christian Leadership Conference recruited black poor for the campaign in Washington. As it had in Martin Luther King's civil rights movement, the basic strength of the campaign came from the black Bible Belt. Passing through the backwoods towns and hamlets of the Deep South, they sang spiritedly, urging others to join them. The sounds of "Oh Freedom" and "Ain't Gonna Let Nobody Turn Me Round" rang out on the main streets and back streets of towns usually bypassed by civil rights workers. Yet beneath the pride, the militancy, the religious fervor, and the excitement, a haunting, almost funereal sadness pervaded the march toward Washington. * "This

* See the sensitive accounts of the march to Washington by Washington *Post* reporter Robert Maynard.

may be America's last chance," Reverend Abernathy said, but many of the poor who so abruptly left their homes to join him may have been thinking, "this *is* our last chance." In the South the black man had become an absolute liability; his cheap labor had been replaced by a cheaper machine. He now had the vote, which white segregationists feared he would use—unless they could starve him out.

The poor people came from the North, too, in restless throngs of snarling young black men whose hatred of society had been forged on bleak city pavements. At least a generation removed from the patient restraint of southern religion, they screamed Action Now, and looked for an excuse to tear down the system that spawned their bitterness. Even in their anger, though, the city people had hopes for this campaign.

From the mountains and foothills of Appalachia, from the deserts and plains of the Southwest, from the dark woods of the far North came the white and Mexican-American poor, their voices mingling with the loud, black cry for help. And from the dusty, hopeless reservations came the sad remnants of this country's first inhabitants— Indians who came to protest their hundred years as virtual prisoners-of-war in America, and to ask that more food and opportunity be shared with their children. Spanish-speaking Americans came, following their volatile leader Reis Tijerina, asking government help in entering the mainstream of life in the United States, and in recapturing grazing land stolen from them so long ago in a great process of white thievery that never made the history books.

Poor people from all over America marched to camp in the plywood tents in the center of Washington and to tell their stories to the nation—a thousand stories that the country needed desperately to hear and learn from. But they came at the wrong time, they did the wrong things, and the country was not listening. Washington was enveloped in chaos.

It rained in Washington from the middle of May until the middle of June, almost one solid month of downpour in the muggy, soggy heat—an agonizing combination to the 3,200 poor people camping on the parkland between the Washington Monument and the Lincoln Memorial. It turned Resurrection City into a stinking quagmire of deep, oozing mud. The mud, always an intimate part of the lives of the rural poor, became important here because the story of the Poor People's Campaign was measured in inches of muck.

After the first few days, most of the Washington reporters stopped writing about the people and why they were there, and concentrated on the mud and the bad tempers of the poor people who were trying to live in it. They wrote about numbers—numbers of fights that broke out during the night, and numbers of arrests made. Ralph David Abernathy protested at a press conference, "The issue is not any kind of dissension or strife that might arise in Resurrection City; the issue is poverty." And his aide, the Reverend Andrew Young, urged reporters who had forgotten their responsibility to focus some attention on the purpose of the campaign. "You have to get used to the fact that poor folks are fussy!"

But the story of dissension, strife between factions, and sights and smells of the muddy village kept pouring into the press rooms of the nation, and everyone soon knew that Washington was irritated by the campaign. Even though hundreds of individual acts of charity eased the hardships of Resurrection City, most of Washington objected to the poor people because they were just plain unsightly. Merchants already hard hit by the April riots panicked at the possible loss of summer business scared away by the shantytown, and Congress considered bill after bill to run the poor people out of the city. Congressional motives received less examination. As SCLC leader Jesse Jackson wisely reflected later, "The press examined minutely the personal behavior of poor people and ignored the collective behavior of Congress."

In the orderly process of government, success of an issue often depends on the skill of its advocates in understanding who holds the key to power on that issue, and how to approach that person in a friendly or persuasive manner. Despite liaison groups organized by sympathetic congressmen, the most powerful committees of Congress were not friendly and were not persuaded. Robert Kennedy, the hunger issue's most popular advocate, was far away, campaigning for the Presidency in the Middle and Far West, and what he had to say about the forgotten poor most often was lost as the press concentrated on the frantic power battle for the Democratic nomination.

The unfriendly Congress evidently gave little thought to the fact that if the poor people had the means to do things the "right way"—to hire a full-time lobbyist to touch the vital pressure points, to provide position papers, inserts for the Congressional Record, steaks and wine for the congressmen—they wouldn't be poor. They were lobbying in the only way they knew how. In the *New Yorker* magazine, Calvin Trillin accurately characterized the overall political and press performance:

"The poor in Resurrection City have come to Washington to show that the poor in America are sick, dirty, disorganized, and powerless—and they are criticized daily for being sick, dirty, disorganized and powerless."

Despite the squabbles, the disorder, the sermonizing, and the fact that the specific needs and desires of the

Negro poor, the Mexican-American poor, and the Indian poor do not necessarily coincide, the various factions were locked into agreement on one issue: Poor people need food, and the food programs do not work.

Reverend Abernathy began to aim his campaign directly at the Department of Agriculture, ordering a round-the-clock demonstration for the sprawling, ugly building that houses the vast bureaucracy, and attempting, time after time, to voice his demands to Freeman.

Finally, Orville Freeman and Ralph David Abernathy faced each other in a sweltering Department of Agriculture conference room, packed with every rain-soaked poor people's campaigner and reporter who could manage to squeeze through the door. Both men mopped at their sweaty faces—Freeman with a white handkerchief, Abernathy with a bright red bandana. Outside, the continuing rain poured in sheets against the windows and added further gloom to an already dismal afternoon.

Abernathy had come to get answers to his demands for improved food programs, and even though two weeks had passed since his "10 days" were up, it was still too soon for Orville Freeman. Both men wanted desperately for this late May meeting to be a success, yet both knew that it would not be. Freeman had sent his written response the previous evening, and they were now going through the ritual of tumultuous public discussion which had become a hallmark of the campaign.

For three weeks, Freeman had waited for a White House answer to the proposed food package, and no answer had come from a President who was as preoccupied with war, inflation, and taxes as he was infuriated at the poor people's street drama.

Annoyed by a bombardment of liberal criticism, which now included the hard-hitting CBS news documentary on hunger (shown May 21), Secretary Freeman wanted to get off the spot but could not move. Finally, he decided on two actions—expanding the limited commodity distribution program by adding fruit juices, scrambled egg mix, canned milk, instant mashed potatoes, canned chicken, and instant hot cereal; and providing food supplements for babies and nursing and expectant mothers. Fearing that President Johnson would veto even this action, the Secretary got *implicit* agreement from White House assistant Joe Califano and Budget Director Zwick, and then went ahead with the $100 million program.

Freeman knew this spare response would not satisfy the demands of the poor, for he belatedly had come to realize that the basic malfunction of the food program was stamps, which cost too much money and provided too little food. He knew also that even beginning this kind of reform would cost at least several hundred million dollars, and that a full reform would cost more than a billion. But above all, he knew that Lyndon Johnson did not seem prepared to spend anything.

In the steamy, crowded conference room, the Secretary of Agriculture was plainly uncomfortable. As questions came popping from every corner, Freeman tried to tell the poor people they might be visiting the wrong man. "I've done about all I can do," he said. "I'm human enough; you might be advised to spend some time with my colleagues."

"Are you telling people they are just waiting, wasting their time?" he was asked.

"I'm next door," he replied. "I'm convenient."

Pressed about the food stamp formula and expansion of the program, the Secretary came closest to telling what he wanted to say, but could not: "The President has this and other matters under consideration." Like most of Washington, Orville Freeman was not attuned to the

168

issue of moral imperative that was being raised by the poor people, but on the other hand, he was misunderstood by them. They saw only his stubborn defense of past progress, and did not know that he secretly was trying to make a political adjustment to their needs. As troubled and pressured as Orville Freeman felt, he could not end the meeting, which droned on and on with a decreasing semblance of order. Ralph David Abernathy also suffered, for he could see by now that—barring some kind of miracle—the tactics of nonviolent militant protest would produce no poverty victories in Washington. The southern minister fell silent, his head bowed, as the poor people screamed at Freeman. Miss Wright and Jesse Jackson, who were better informed on the issues than Abernathy was, continued their futile debate—futile because Freeman was powerless to act, and because the campaign itself did not contain the dynamics for success in Washington.

As he sat slumped in a wooden chair in the Agriculture Department, Abernathy reflected how different had been the results in Selma and Birmingham, where the civil rights movement was bloodied and brutalized, but produced great legislative victories. He was now using the same confrontation tactics that just three years before had brought waves of sympathy from the North, but this time he sought to evoke the national conscience about national conditions which result in poverty all across America—not merely about decaying southern social and political structures. He was calling on the nation to re-order its economic priorities, and no brutal southern sheriff was going to get the job done for him.

Abernathy had just realized that when a Negro was bloodied by dogs in Birmingham for the right to sit in a restaurant, the white northerner was a sympathetic ally.

When the same Negro, who never had been able to afford that hard-won southern right, tried to dramatize his hunger in Washington, the same white northerner disapproved. It was easy enough to blame a southerner for barring his restaurant door, and it cost nothing to suggest remedies; but who was the northern white man to blame for nationwide hunger, except himself, and who would have to pay for its cure?

In the early evening, the inconclusive meeting came to an end. It was the last time Freeman and Abernathy would meet during the campaign. Little of this drama was reported except what the shortsighted press was able to make out of mud, misery, and squabbling. The public tired of hearing about the noisy shouting matches. They were being asked to think why some citizens were hungry, dirty, ill-fed, and ill-housed, and to look at them in all their poorness walking through the nation's capital.

Public annoyance at these confrontation tactics was now reflected in the Harris poll, which showed 61 percent of white America disapproving of the campaign. And if the Poor People's Campaign did not stir the nation's conscience at the beginning it certainly was doomed after the first rock was thrown at the Supreme Court.

During a May 29 demonstration at the Supreme Court building, several rocks crashed through basement windows. It was possible but not proven that the rocks had been thrown by persons from Resurrection City. On the positive side that same day, the Senate produced one of the few legislative victories of the campaign, and a dramatic hearing about human need stirred a Senate committee. Press treatment of these three events tells much about the inability of the Poor People's Campaign to reach the American people.

The rock-throwing incident produced banner headlines

in newspapers across the country. The facts were unclear about responsibility for the broken windows as campaign marshals helped restore order, and the turmoil at the court was brief. Few stories devoted more than a sentence to the reason for the protest demonstration—a Court decision upholding Washington state regulations barring Indians from net fishing in their traditional fishing grounds. But the news for the day focused on the visual drama in the Capital, not on the plight of America's first citizens trying desperately to cling to their age-old means of nutrition and survival.

Little or no attention was paid to the hard-won fight across the street at the United States Senate, where Senator Jacob Javits' amendment to release $227 million of Section 32 funds for use to feed the hungry was passed in a breathtaking 31–30 vote.*

But the most meaningful event of the day for poor, hungry Americans was virtually a non-event, because most of the nation's press ignored it. Attorney Marian Wright, seeking out individual poor people in Resurrection City, had structured a presentation to reveal every conceivable viewpoint about hunger, and about the operation of government food programs. She brought 15 people to the huge hearing room in the basement of the New Senate Office Building, and they all spoke from the heart, with no prepared words, no coaching from advisers.

Mrs. Lupe Martinez from Denver, Colorado, who paid $94 of her $200 monthly income to purchase food stamps, protested about the program's prohibition against buying soap. "I am poor but I do like to get down on my knees and live the clean way. It is kind of hard to do when you don't have money left over to buy detergents."

* The Javits proposal died from inaction in the House of Representatives.

A high school dropout from Denver told how it felt to use a different-colored card for a reduced price lunch. "When you hand the card to the cashier, people would look at you. You feel low. It should not be like that. We should not have certain colors to separate us; like one rich, one poor, something like that."

Mrs. Tina Kruger, a strong-willed white woman from Hidalgo County, Texas, told how she adopted two starving infants who were handed to her by their penniless migrant mothers, each with the plea, "Here, you take this baby home because I have nothing to feed him. He is dying of starvation and I do not want him to die in my home."

Mrs. Ellis Blackhorse, an elderly Indian from Idaho Spring, South Dakota, explained to the senators that she is a diabetic who cannot live on the starchy foods of a commodity program diet, and has no source of income to supplement it.

Representing the black poor of Mississippi, Mrs. Myrtle Brown explained how a woman with $68 monthly income could afford to pay neither the $28 monthly to participate in the food stamp program nor the 25 cents apiece daily for each of her five children to participate in the school lunch program. At noontime the five children walk a mile to and from school in hopes of lunch. "Some days they come and find me with food," she said. "Some days they come and don't find me with anything."

Senator Jennings Randolph, the affable West Virginia Democrat, could hardly believe Mrs. Jose Williams' tale of the Mississippi plantation owner who loaned her $22 to buy food stamps until her welfare check came in and demanded repayment with $28 worth of stamps, which he apparently exchanged for cash at a relative's grocery store. "This is an abominable practice," said Senator Randolph. "It is an abominable practice and should be checked out." If Senator Randolph and his colleagues had even scratched the politics of hunger in the Deep South, they would have known that hundreds of plantation owners traditionally charged interest when they advanced survival money to their black serfs.

Many of the most important human facts about the politics of hunger were laid bare at that Senate hearing, but the country was not listening.

On June 6 Senator Robert F. Kennedy was murdered in Los Angeles and the faint flicker of hopeful light went out in Resurrection City. The press descended in mass to test the emotions of the poor at the death of their only white hero. The reporters expected anguished wailing, wondered why it wasn't there, and were resented by the poor for wondering. For the poor, the murder was barely surprising. From their viewpoint, it was almost a certainty now that all the leaders who tried to help them would be murdered. One more good man was dead, and many of the poor were too drained of emotion even to cry. They would neither perform nor riot—to the relief of Washington officialdom who expected a repeat of the rioting following Dr. King's death. Abernathy quietly led a delegation to the funeral at Arlington cemetery and then they walked back across Memorial Bridge to the mud of Resurrection City, the dream that had become just one more nightmare.

As things went from bad to worse, Abernathy and his lieutenants started looking for a way out. Working desperately to salvage some tangible gain for poor Americans before the encampment was torn down by an angry, harassed government, the campaign's friends tried to achieve at least some meaningful reforms by Solidarity Day, June 19. The "June 'teenth," anniversary of the

Emancipation Proclamation, might stimulate a spark of national conscience, as thousands of Americans from all over the country planned to join the Resurrection City residents in a one-day demonstration of support. Hopefully, Solidarity Day would repeat the successful 1963 March on Washington, when Martin Luther King's impassioned oratory had stirred the nation. Several high Johnson Administration officials shared that hope and they frantically worked to produce a miracle for Solidarity Day.

While 75 demonstrators shouted beneath his second-floor window, "We want food . . . We want freedom . . . We want Freeman!" Agriculture Undersecretary John Schnittker launched a new effort to develop a legislative package for the President. Together with Budget Bureau official Bernard Gladieux, Undersecretary Schnittker (a Robert Kennedy intimate who had privately sought to help throughout the Poor People's Campaign) designed a new program to provide the poor with more food stamps at less cost. But when Schnittker contacted the White House with the new plan, word came back "Nothing doing while the tax bill is pending!"

Seeking out old friends who had helped before, legislative adviser Marian Wright and the Reverend Jesse Jackson, leader of the Southern Christian Leadership Conference's highly successful Chicago program, met with aides of Vice President Hubert Humphrey. They explained to sympathetic John Stewart and William Welsh that the poor people would end the encampment if the President would only make reforms in the food aid programs. They asked that the reforms be announced on Solidarity Day.

After a briefing by Stewart, Humphrey telephoned President Johnson that night (June 11) to tell him the campaign could be terminated on very reasonable terms. Following up with a memorandum to the President the next day, Humphrey emphasized: "The key is a package dealing with hunger and food. . . . A major breakthrough here—one which could be defended publicly on the sound humanitarian basis of feeding hungry people—would be interpreted by the SCLC leadership as an honorable basis of ending the Campaign." The only other requirements were that the Administration seek repeal of the congressionally imposed welfare freeze, announce support for the concept of a public service employment bill, and support the concept of greater participation by the poor in the planning and implementation of programs affecting them. Humphrey urged that such a program "could be the device for bringing the Poor People's Campaign to a constructive and honorable end with Resurrection City dismantled by June 23."

"From the Administration's point of view," Humphrey wrote, "the settlement could be cast in a totally affirmative fashion. 'We are acting to see that no American goes to bed hungry; we are acting to insure that every American who wants to work and is able to work has a job.' This posture largely avoids the charge that we were responding to intimidation and undue pressure."

Humphrey concluded that such a settlement "would strengthen the hand of responsible Negro leaders, meet the most urgent needs of hunger and jobs, and add to the Administration's already considerable accomplishments in these areas." Abernathy, attempting to carry out his end of a negotiated settlement, scaled down his demands to match this list. His food program now was identical to the one Johnson's own aides had recommended to the President weeks earlier.

Although Vice President Humphrey offered his services

175

as mediator, and was supported in his plan by Attorney General Ramsey Clark (to whom President Johnson had assigned responsibility for the Poor People's Campaign), it is doubtful that the President ever read Humphrey's message. The memo was stopped en route by White House aide Harry McPherson, who believed that President Johnson would react unfavorably. The President already had been pressured too hard on food aid and on the Poor People's Campaign, he said. Judging from the President's outburst at Orville Freeman the same day as the Humphrey memo, McPherson had correctly sensed Johnson's mood.

Freeman, again acting without Presidential clearance but with the knowledge of White House aide Califano, decided to support 108 liberal congressmen * who by this time had asked for an unlimited authorization for the food stamp program. Testifying before the House Agriculture Committee in defense of the food stamp program, Freeman asked for the unlimited authorization. The Secretary reasoned that he would thus satisfy the liberals without actually committing the President to more spending, since an appropriations bill still would be needed to implement an increase in actual food stamp funds. Within seconds after Freeman uttered the word "unlimited," Poage and ranking Republican Page Belcher of Oklahoma snarled that this didn't sound like the same administration that had just promised to cut $6 billion in spending. One Agriculture Committee member promptly telephoned these sentiments to the White House and a furi-

* Representative Leonor Sullivan, Agriculture Department officials and traditional Democratic leaders worked up the petition which became part of another trade with southerners, permitting the food stamp expansion in return for an extension of the farm subsidy program.

ous Lyndon Johnson told Freeman his completely un-authorized statement had endangered the tax bill.

The tax increase was scheduled for a final vote in the House the afternoon following Solidarity Day, and Lyndon Johnson was not about to risk last-minute defeat by unveiling a new spending plan or by giving anything to the unruly demonstrators.

Despite protests from the District of Columbia Appropriations Subcommittee, the campers' permit was extended for one week, to allow for Solidarity Day, and on June 19, more than a hundred thousand middle-class Americans joined Resurrection City residents and marched from the Capitol to the Lincoln Memorial. The throng stood united in front of Abraham Lincoln's statue, remembering a happier occasion there five years earlier, when Dr. Martin Luther King, Jr., had told of his dream for a better America. This time they received no word of support from the White House.

The next day Congress finally passed the tax increase with its $6 billion dollar spending slash, and Washington police used tear gas to rout 300 demonstrators from an attempted sit-in in the street beside the Department of Agriculture.

Four days later, a thousand heavily armed policemen captured a nearly deserted Resurrection City, while its few hundred remaining inhabitants purposely violated the off-limits grounds of the United States Capitol. They concluded their unsuccessful campaign with their own arrests. Ralph David Abernathy attempted to make one last plea to Freeman, met briefly with his executive assistant, then went to the Capitol to be arrested with his followers.

If the Poor People's Campaign had begun with hopes that the nation's conscience could be aroused, it ended as a disaster, with even its leaders agreeing that the encampment on the Mall had been a mistake. A few substantial reforms in the administration of federal programs had been won, but the poor people had failed to touch the soul of the country, and they knew it. Most of those remaining finished their jail terms and started home, convinced that the nation did not care.

By that time, however, a host of Washington officials *did* care strongly about food program reform. Some had actually been moved by the Poor People's Campaign. Only hours after the tax bill cleared conference, the men who cared started back toward the President with their new proposals. With the tax bill finally out of the way they thought President Johnson would be sure to favor their plans.

Drafted by Agriculture Undersecretary Schnittker, the new hunger program was shaped into a memorandum from Secretary Freeman to President Johnson, beginning: "To meet the highest priority food needs in the next 12 months will require adding $300–400 million to the food program in the 1969 budget. *This will not end hunger in the U.S., but it will make a big down payment on a program to end hunger shortly.*"

Freeman went on to explain that legislative actions to carry out such a program were well along in Congress, but he also offered the President an alternate $145 million program, merely to pay for the commitments Agriculture already had made to the Poor People's Campaign. The main point of the memo, however, was a strong recommendation for a $410 million program reforming the food stamp formula and improving food assistance to poor school children.

Enthusiastic White House aides, including the President's close adviser Charles Murphy, grabbed the memo and escalated Freeman's proposal into a $465 million program for 1969, and a three-year, $2-billion commitment which would "guarantee every American freedom from starvation and serious malnutrition." Because Murphy, Vice President Humphrey, and others close to him had been urging him to take another look at the food program, President Johnson consented to listen to the proposal, and told Joe Califano to call a meeting.

At 5:30 p.m. on June 28, 1968, Agriculture Secretary Freeman, Budget Director Zwick, and White House assistants Murphy, Califano, Pierson, and James Gaither filed into the President's oval office, confident that Johnson would now act positively on food for the hungry poor. Earlier in the day, the Chief Executive had signed the tax bill; now, finally, he could devote his attention to other domestic matters. So, while his staff waited expectantly, President Johnson glanced for the first time at a simply outlined four-page memo in which Califano had described the proposal.

Halfway down the second page, the Presidential eyes focused on the heading "Actions by Freeman" and the explanation: "Merely to carry out the commitments recently made by Secretary Freeman to improve the commodity distribution and food stamp programs in fiscal 1969 would require $145 million over the 1969 budget." Lyndon B. Johnson looked up at Orville Freeman, frowned, and exploded.

"A hundred and forty-five million dollars—I never authorized you to do that!" the President raged. "Don't you realize that I have just signed a tax bill promising to cut spending by *six billion dollars?*"

Freeman was totally taken aback by Johnson's latest tirade. The Secretary had announced the improvements in the commodity program more than a month earlier and had made repeated references to them without repercussions from the Chief Executive. Orville Freeman turned toward Califano and said, "Joe cleared it."

When Califano nodded his head in agreement, the President turned his anger toward Budget Director Zwick, whose chief function is to safeguard the Presidential budget.

"I didn't clear it but I was aware of it," Zwick said nervously. "Joe cleared it and we thought he was speaking for you."

Johnson fumed that he now was compelled to reduce spending and wasn't going to start that exercise by adding almost half a billion dollars to the budget.

Freeman attempted to explain that food aid no longer was an isolated legislative program but now was tied together politically with a four-year extension of the farm program. "Liberal and southern Democrats already are working together as they did in 1964 to trade support on measures for an expanded food stamp program and for continued farm price supports," he said. But President Johnson ended the meeting abruptly, ordering Califano to revise the plan downward to meet only minimum requirements, and gruffly told Freeman to send him a memorandum clarifying the political situation on Capitol Hill.

An agitated Orville Freeman returned to his office. For more than a year he had lived with intense conflicting pressures on the food issue. When he had first accepted the Cabinet job, his principal political assignment from President Kennedy, and later from President Johnson, had been to cajole Southern conservatives like Ellender, Poage, and Whitten to win necessary agricultural programs and to keep "the farm problem" off the President's back. Secretary Freeman had carried out his assignment well, with hundreds of hours spent carefully catering to the super-conservative personalities of men like Ellender and Whitten. Civil rights and poverty had been given low priorities for him in those early years, making it difficult to switch gears when these issues finally focused on his department in the late 1960s. He had taken excessive criticism from liberals for 16 months, even though he now, at last, favored reform and the criticism belonged at the doorstep of the White House.

When he reached his own office Orville Freeman called in his secretary and hastily dictated for the President an emotion-charged memorandum which revealed a great deal about the Agriculture Secretary and his views on both the politics of hunger and Lyndon Johnson.

"The current attack on the Administration alleging callousness and incompetence in the face of widespread hunger and malnutrition is the most difficult problem to handle for me since the Billie Sol Estes case," [*] Freeman began. "In the Billie Sol Estes case the effort was solely to destroy the Administration. This is part of the current pattern, but also the present attacks hope to capture public attention and support so that other objectives they have in the war on poverty can be accomplished."

Although he alleged that the issue had been raised from such conspiratorial motives, Freeman told the President that hunger was a very real problem, one he had seen with his own eyes. Further, he dictated, it was now getting a strong, emotional dose of public attention because of the Citizens' Board of Inquiry and the school lunch reports, the CBS television program, and "the tactics and efforts of the so-called poor people."

[*] Estes used Texas Democratic and Washington Agriculture Department connections to further moneymaking schemes for which he was indicted and convicted in federal court.

Although he was still receiving thousands of critical letters as a result of the "shockingly irresponsible CBS program," Freeman said "my counterattack [against the program] had been important." *

"The counterattack has given us at least a sounding board, for my charges have captured attention and some of the real facts are coming to public attention," Freeman wrote. "In the process, I believe people will become aware of all the things we have done and are doing to meet the food requirements of the needy."

In his attempt to justify the actions which brought on the Presidential tongue-lashing, Freeman wrote a small essay on the politics of hunger. "Where I have felt it necessary," he said, "I have yielded a bit and liberalized the program. Otherwise, in my best judgment, we would have been painted into a very tight corner and made to look callous and indifferent. . . . I can assure you in making some concessions where the use of Section 32 funds are concerned, I was not acting counter to the President's intentions as I understood them at that time.

"At the same time I have made some concessions in the programs where we were most vulnerable if we stood hard and yielded not at all, I have stood fast on other points. I won't relate them all. Free food stamps for the lowest income group is an example. There are many others where I have simply said no. This firmness has come through to the public.

* Freeman publicly condemned the CBS program for its very minor factual inaccuracies and its failure to praise what he considered to be improvements in the food programs. Freeman failed to see or to admit that the primary purpose of this powerful program was to show that hunger existed in America, despite federal food programs. Columnist Carl Rowan said Freeman could have better used his anger in public criticism of the Jamie Whittens of Congress.

182

"At least, I find many people who write or come to me and say thank goodness you are standing firm and not letting this ragtail, bobtailed group of so-called 'Poor People' push you around. What I have tried to do is hold to the middle ground so that people around the nation sensitive to the hunger and malnutrition problem will not feel that the Administration has been completely callous, cold, and heartless. At the same time I have tried hard to avoid an image of being intimidated or weak-kneed.

"I hopefully recommend that you decide on a generous food package and send a special message to the Congress soon. . . ."

With this message, the food issue headed back on one of its many trips to President Johnson's desk.

White House aides Califano, Gaither, and Murphy, along with officials at the Budget Bureau and Agriculture Department worked over the week-end of June 29–30, revising the food program so they could get it back to the President on Monday.

At 6 p.m. Monday, July 1, 1968, Califano sent into the President a two-and-a-half page memorandum concisely outlining a scaled-down $285 million food program he said had been agreed to by Freeman, Zwick, Gaither, Pierson, Murphy, and himself. About one-half the money would be used to meet commitments made by Freeman to the poor people and to counties which had been promised the food program. But the new food package's most important ingredient was a $95 million plan to begin liberalizing the food stamp program for families with between $30 and $170 monthly income.

If another meeting were necessary, Califano suggested, it should be held the next day because "it would be important to move quickly after the [congressional] recess to get the necessary legislative action."

Knowing that Lyndon Johnson always liked "to keep his options open," Califano—after strongly urging action—offered three options for the President's personal check mark. These were: "Set up meeting with Zwick, Murphy, and Gaither tomorrow. Proceed with drafting of the message [to Congress]. See me."

The President read Califano's memo and scrawled a big check mark by the option, "See me."

"Give me some reasons why I should approve this program," President Johnson told Califano. The assistant argued that the Administration had made commitments and would look bad in not keeping them.

"You say I've made a commitment," the President said. "Get me the words of that commitment."

Califano pointed out that in signing the Food Stamp Act in 1967 the President had pledged that he would place a food program in each of the nation's 1,000 poorest counties which lacked one. That had led to "Project 331," * and now some of the extra food stamp money was needed to start programs in about 50 of these counties.

"I didn't know that commitment was going to cost money," Johnson snapped. "The next time you send me a commitment, let me know how much it is going to cost." (President Johnson made no decision on the food program but he did give Joe Califano a new "extra duty" assignment: whenever a speech draft was prepared for the President, Califano had to examine it carefully and note on it whether it committed the President to any

* President Johnson vowed to place a food program in each of the 331 poorest counties (out of the 1,000 lowest in per capita income) that did not already have a food program. This approach did not touch the poor in counties where poverty was masked statistically by the affluence of many other residents.

184

spending. This punishment lasted for about a week, until President Johnson's mind turned to other matters.)

After the new proposal lay dormant for several days, Vice President Humphrey personally appealed for approval of the food plan, now that the tax increase bill was safely enacted.

"I've given my word to Congress [on the spending cut]," Johnson replied in turning down Humphrey's entreaty. "If you can get Congress to do something, fine. But we've made a commitment. We've talked to Ellender, Poage, and Whitten. I'm not going to be the one to break that agreement. That's what they're waiting for up there. If I break the agreement, we'll never get anything else through Congress."

No one close to the President is quite certain what agreements he made with whom, or whether he actually promised southern reactionaries that he would not propose broad changes in food programs. The hard-won combination tax increase and appropriation reduction bill certainly made no such commitment. Its only promise was to reduce spending somewhere, and the President had all the options of deciding where. The matter is not clarified by the fact that, about this same time, President Johnson went before the weekly meeting of the government's congressional liaison officers and told them not to be concerned about emasculation of domestic programs.

"Now, don't any of you bleeding hearts worry," he told them. "Lady Bird and Luci and Lynda have already got on to me about not cutting education and health. I'm not going to get them mad. We'll make the reductions in the SST, the space program, and some military construction spending, and then you watch Congress. They'll put the money right back in."

Although Humphrey was now frantically involved in his bid for the Presidential nomination, the Vice President tried one last device to persuade the President. Both his wife Muriel and Mrs. Arthur Krim, wife of the film magnate and chief Presidential fund raiser, were active members of the President's Commission on Mental Retardation and both were concerned about studies showing the possible effects of malnutrition on infant mental development. He knew the President was fond of Mathilda Krim, and thought that perhaps she could get through to him. Unable to reach her on the telephone, Humphrey did something he usually carefully avoided—he put into written form a criticism of President Lyndon Johnson.

"It is just intolerable to me that there is such a problem of malnutrition and undernourishment in the United States, with our great agricultural production. It hurts the children the most, and they are the least able to bear it," he wrote to Mathilda Krim.

"Through it all, there are ways the President could have helped—in approving some of Orville Freeman's budget requests, in supporting legislation on the Hill, and suggesting administrative change—but he has not. The thought came that you might be the person who could say a word or two to encourage him to move more conclusively to solve this hunger problem.

"Someone associated with the health field could bring to him a new point of view. So many people have talked about hunger from the poverty and racial perspective that it has tended to blur the sheer physical impact of hunger. . . . We need to put the hunger issue aside from special interests and see it as the human interest it is."

Mathilda Krim telephoned the President in Texas to ask his help in fighting hunger, but Johnson still refused to act.

During the last months of the Johnson Administration, Orville Freeman, White House aides, and even the normally conservative Budget Bureau doggedly continued bringing the President plans to make a national commitment against hunger.

When a final supplemental appropriations bill was being prepared in the last days of the 90th Congress, Califano and Budget Director Zwick urged the President to seek the full $90 million of increased food stamp appropriations which Congress had authorized, even without backing from the White House.

"How can I single food out, when education and all these other programs also need money?"

"Because Congress has authorized it," the President was told.

"Well, they won't fund it. They'll leave me holding the bag," the President said. "It's out of the question. Forget it."

Then, two days later, at a meeting with the various congressional appropriations chairmen, the President apparently had a sudden change of heart, and in a move which surprised everyone concerned, asked them for the money. But it was late in the day. Congress did approve $55 million for the food stamp program, but this amount barely covered the commitments Agriculture had made to counties almost a year before.

When it came time for him to sign the Food Stamp Extension Bill, Budget Bureau and White House aides tried to get President Johnson to establish a Food and Nutrition Council and to make at least a verbal commitment to end hunger. The proposed text would have clearly stated the problem and what needed to be done. The text was discarded by the President.

Although the President had said "no" about as many

times and in as many ways a man could, Administration insiders persisted in the belief that he would face this problem before he left office. "Wait for Lyndon Johnson's last budget and State of the Union message," they kept saying.

With such thoughts in mind Agriculture Secretary Freeman went to the White House after the election in November for one last try at the food issue.

"Mr. President," he argued. "This is our last chance. You've had all these terrible restrictions and pressures. Why not now, for once in eight years, fund a budget that makes up the Great Society. I'd like you to put in a budget that I believe in and you believe in. Let Nixon cut it."

Using yet another line of reasoning, Johnson now told Freeman, "I just don't know about these programs. Food comes and food goes. You don't get anything for it. Education and job training get more for the money."

Because the President appeared so completely negative on the issue, Freeman sent him a final memorandum, saying he would be misunderstood if he did not at least request the full $340 million food stamp authorization. In the end, Freeman was authorized to commit a program, including quite minor food stamp reform, that would cost the Nixon Administration $340 million in fiscal 1970 unless Nixon tried to change signals. President Johnson's final argument, and perhaps the best of many he used during the year, was that he should not make decisions for the new administration.

On at least 12 specific occasions his aides and Cabinet officers had recommended food aid reform and Lyndon Johnson had said "no." None of those closest to his thinking and decision-making are certain what really stopped the President on the issue of hunger and malnutrition in America. They know only that the President's motives were often complex, even conflicting. When he turned down the Task Force reports in 1966 and 1967, the President was skeptical about the existence of a little-publicized problem, and perhaps he was in this no different from most Americans. But this was the particular type of problem that usually appealed personally to Lyndon Johnson. He liked tackling and quickly solving basic problems involving human beings—and hunger certainly met this criterion.

He had legitimate concern about moving on the hunger issue while the tax bill was hanging in the balance with conservative Wilbur Mills. On these grounds, any criticism of the President must go right to the issue of the Vietnam war itself and to the government's sense of national priorities. As the war expanded and became increasingly more expensive, Johnson felt strongly that fund-raising and anti-inflationary measures had top priority. Once the tax bill passed, however, other reasons must be found to explain the President's inaction. He had selected many other issues from congressional proponents and made them his own, but perhaps in this case, he, like Jamie Whitten, saw a Kennedy maneuver. He disliked Robert Kennedy intensely and this had been a Kennedy issue from the outset.

There is no doubt that Lyndon Johnson believed he was being pushed and, if there was one thing he resented, it was having other people make up his mind for him. His fury at Freeman for making overtures to the poor people and asking Congress for an unlimited food stamp authorization convinced his advisers that Johnson felt others were trying to commit him. He fumed repeatedly about Freeman's actions in increasing the cost of the commodity program and recommending a larger food stamp program. He suspected that Freeman, Murphy, Zwick,

Califano, and others on his own staff were making decisions behind his back. And in several instances they almost were—out of a sense of desperate frustration to get a decision from him.

"What can we do to get the President to act?" a Humphrey aide asked Presidential assistant Harry McPherson. "You might stop pushing him," McPherson replied. "He doesn't like it."

The tactics of the Poor People's Campaign were opposed by public opinion, and poll-watcher Johnson perhaps didn't want to appear pushed into action by what even Orville Freeman called a "ragtailed, bobtailed group."

Did Lyndon Johnson disapprove of food programs because "you don't get anything for it?" According to a close White House aide, this comment indicated Johnson's strong dislike of food aid as "welfare," while the President's own populist thinking supported programs which provided opportunity. If this were the key to the President's negative behavior, it ignored the fact that an infant crippled by malnutrition could never be helped by any amount of education or job training.

At one point, Johnson deferred action by contending that Congress would not approve food stamp reform. If he truly believed this, the master congressional politician had not studied 1968 congressional action on the issue. Majorities in both the House and the Senate had approved major food program expenditures and reforms, but the efforts could not be coordinated without full Presidential backing. There is little doubt that Congress would have taken major steps forward on the hunger issue in 1968 if Lyndon Johnson had only lent his support.

Perhaps in the end, President Lyndon Johnson, like many of us in America, consciously and unconsciously practiced the politics of ignorance. His pride was great and it was difficult for him to admit, after five years of trying hard to build a Great Society, that a most basic problem of poverty had not even been examined, much less solved.

If President Johnson failed completely to confront the *full* hunger and malnutrition issue during his term in office, at least he contributed toward progress in improving the government's food aid programs. Specific programs aimed at providing food for the poor rose from $173 million in the last year of the Eisenhower administration to $403 million in fiscal 1968 and $655 million in fiscal 1969. Beginning with President Kennedy's first executive order, the two successive Democratic administrations did start slowly converting surplus disposal programs into human food programs.

Major strides were taken in 1968, principally because liberals in Congress finally followed the early leaders and fought to get programs through. The initial efforts of Senators Kennedy, Clark, Mondale, Javits, and McGovern and Congressmen Foley, Goodell, and Quie eventually involved most liberal-to-moderate members of both political parties. These men attempted with some success to roll over the opposition of the Poages and Whittens, even though the President would not. The results were an improved commodity distribution program, a $43 million appropriation to provide free or reduced priced meals to needy children, the bare beginnings of a reformed food stamp program that really serves the poor, and the creation of the Senate Select Committee which would probe the politics of hunger in 1969.

The hunger effort of 1968 really ended, though, with the breakup of Resurrection City and the few congressional breakthroughs for better food programs. When the poor people had started their mule train from Mississippi, campaign leader Hosea Williams had looked up at white bystanders watching the march and told them, "You're glad to see these niggers leaving Mississippi but you ain't gonna be glad to see these niggers coming back!"

Indeed, many of the black poor who started out on the campaign had hoped to find some miraculous escape in Washington. But by the time they held their last meeting with Secretary Freeman, their sad thoughts turned to "back home."

A Mrs. Brooks from Sunflower County, Mississippi, protested that she can't afford to spend $56 monthly for food stamps, and "can't get my children school lunches with food stamps."

"There's plenty of food," Freeman answered, "the problem sometimes is with the local people."

"In Sunflower County, Senator Eastland is the local people," someone shouted from the back of the room.

"Admit that Eastland is a racist," someone else yelled.

"I can't correct the southern mentality," Freeman replied.

"Will you go with Mrs. Brooks to Sunflower County?" someone shouted.

Freeman did not answer.

"We're here in Washington and we'll die here before we go back to that," Mrs. Brooks said.

Despite her desperation and her dreams, the camp was closed and Mrs. Brooks had to go home.

# CHAPTER XI

# The Priorities of Richard Nixon

LATE IN THE AFTERNOON OF MAY 6, 1969, PRESI-
dent Richard M. Nixon surprised most of official Washington by asking Congress for one billion dollars to reform the food programs. Just two days earlier, the new
administration had had no plans for alleviating hunger
in America. Round three in the politics of hunger is the
story of how and why the President acted.

Even if the Nixon proposal were adopted, the billion
dollars would fall short of an adequate program, and
many hungry children would have to wait at least another
year for help. The President asked for only a $270 million
increase for fiscal 1970, and an additional $1 billion for
1971.

But a significant turning point in the politics of hunger
was reached when an American President publicly acknowledged that millions of poor Americans suffer from

*193*

inadequate nutrition, and vowed to do something about it. "That hunger and malnutrition should persist in a land such as ours is embarrassing and intolerable," President Nixon said. "More is at stake here than the health and well-being of 16 million American citizens who will be aided by these programs. Something like the very honor of American democracy is involved."

Nixon's plan called for providing the poor with sufficient food stamps for an adequate diet and for lowering the cost of stamps toward a level the poor might be able to afford. Former President Johnson had turned down similar plans on a dozen occasions, but the politics of hunger were shifting rapidly in the early months of 1969.

During his campaign for the Presidency, Richard Nixon had referred only once to the possibility that many Americans lack adequate food. That passing reference mainly reflected the efforts of citizen lobbyist Robert Choate to insert food aid reform into the campaign. Had Robert Kennedy lived, hunger might have become a campaign issue. It was not, however, and Nixon felt no pressure to make it one, especially as Choate had been able to produce only token commitments from opponents Hubert Humphrey, Eugene McCarthy, and Nelson Rockefeller. The Nixon campaign was pitched to a political majority which he referred to as "forgotten Americans"—a silent, law-abiding, backlash-prone white middle class that shied away from the problems of black minorities in particular, and from those of the poor in general. Seldom so much as mentioning the problems of poverty, Candidate Nixon at one point warned Congress not to be pressured into accepting the demands of the Poor People's Campaign. The chief demand was to feed the hungry poor.

Against this background of apparent indifference, the Washington food aid reformers gloomily predicted that food aid would receive little attention from still another President. Their pessimism was premature, however, because it ignored a basic political reality: Demands of the Presidency are far more complex than those of campaign politics. Following each national election, the country first must wait innocently to see if the newly elected Chief Executive will carry out his campaign pledges; then it must watch him deal with entirely different issues—problems he may have ignored completely during the campaign. Candidate Nixon had not reckoned on the political pressures built up by hunger.

Two days after President Nixon took office, the food program reformers received the kind of information they had been waiting for—authoritative scientific proof of hunger and malnutrition in America. Produced by the National Nutrition Survey, a study ordered as one result of a 1967 legislative victory for the hunger issue, the initial findings of the first federal investigation into the nutritional health of the American poor gave Congress and the Nixon Administration some of the "hard" numbers a skeptical Lyndon Johnson had demanded.

Dr. Arnold Schaefer, the nutrition survey director, testified before the Senate Select Committee on Nutrition, which had been created by a 1968 legislative victory. The scientist revealed statistics that immediately added a new dimension to the politics of hunger. Whereas the testimony of Robert Kennedy, the Field Foundation doctors, *Hunger USA*, and the poor themselves had been greeted with disbelief and hostility, the doubters now were confronted with that kind of evidence this nation worships— truths found in test tubes and tabulated by computers.

Noting that the nutritional deficiencies found among poor Americans remarkably resembled those found in populations of the world's least developed countries, Dr.

195

Schaefer reported: "Our studies to date clearly indicate that there is malnutrition—and in our opinion it occurs in an unexpectedly large proportion of our sample population!"

Without Arnold Schaefer's tenacity, there would have been no survey results to influence the politics of hunger. After conducting 31 nutrition studies in undeveloped countries as part of the foreign aid and defense effort, Schaefer was incredulous that the United States government seemed content to know more about the health of children in distant lands than of those in America. The tough, bantamweight biochemist fought the Health, Education, and Welfare bureaucracy for three years to get money for the American nutrition survey. Of the small group of key food aid reformers, only Schaefer came from the middle ranks of the federal bureaucracy. In marked contrast to most bureaucrats, he was willing to risk the displeasure of his bosses, and his job, to obtain his objective.

Schaefer's most disturbing data concerned malnutrition in young children, the very group most susceptible to permanent harmful effects from lack of proper food. He found poverty children lagging from six months to two-and-a-half years behind their peers in physical development; 34 percent were badly anemic; 33 percent suffered severe shortage of Vitamin A (of which fortified milk is a primary source); and 16 percent lacked adequate amounts of Vitamin C.

A week later, a highly respected pediatrician from the National Institutes of Health, Dr. Charles Upton Lowe, spelled out the effects that hunger can have on babies. "It is our conviction that nutrition is the key to the normal development of children," Dr. Lowe told the same Senate Select Committee, as he described the vicious, crushing role of malnutrition in infant mortality, prematurity, and mental retardation. In direct, powerful language, he was translating scientific findings into human concerns.

These new medical facts, set forth by Dr. Schaefer and explained by Dr. Lowe, became front-page news which did not escape the attention of the new President. Following a briefing by Health, Education, and Welfare Secretary Robert Finch, President Nixon made a strong statement on the hunger issue in a mid-February speech to HEW employees, and another at the Agriculture Department.

In his appeal to the President, Finch, in turn, had been briefed by the indefatigable Robert Choate. During the first few months of the Nixon administration, Choate conducted a virtual one-man college on hunger, eagerly making his way into offices of the new executives, attempting to educate and stimulate them into action. With a flourish of showmanship and hard-sell business technique, Choate captured Finch's interest by displaying an assortment of highly fortified foods. At his first meeting with White House Urban Affairs Adviser Daniel Patrick Moynihan, Choate burst into his office, announcing that the food stamp plan "amounts to criminal extortion of the poor."

"Don't tell me things like that," shot back a skeptical Moynihan. Choate then laid out the food stamp tables, showing Moynihan how much money persons with low incomes must pay. He made his point.

Choate moved in and out of the Administration, taking an official role as a consultant to the Department of Health, Education, and Welfare when he thought being "inside" was the most effective way to influence the new officials, resigning and again assuming the role of a public critic when he became convinced Nixon would not act.

*197*

Although he usually referred to himself as a "liberal Republican businessman," Choate's style more closely approached that of consumer crusader Ralph Nader. His commitment was to action on the hunger issue, and any political alliances that moved him toward that goal were welcome.

President Nixon mentioned Choate's contribution in his February speech at the Health, Education, and Welfare Department. Other impromptu remarks followed, drawing the President into the hunger issue. Because the initial words of new Presidents are closely noted, that speech began to commit his Administration. But the focal point for hunger remained on Capitol Hill.

Another significant breakthrough—not measurable in statistical terms—came on February 19. Democratic Senator Ernest F. Hollings of South Carolina broke the bonds of southern tradition by stating that the southern white man had lied about black poverty, and had always practiced the politics of ignorance. "There is hunger in South Carolina," tall, silver-haired Fritz Hollings began telling the Senate Select Committee, and in his deep Charleston voice described how things really were, and always had been, in the South. Portraying the lives of countless poor, with names and faces, the southern senator told of a vicious circle of poverty that produces illness, school dropouts, lack of skills, and eventually, theft for food and survival.

"How many is the time that my friends have pointed a finger and said, 'Look at that dumb Negro!'" said Hollings. "The charge is too often accurate. He is dumb, because we have denied him food. Dumb in infancy, he has been blighted for life.

"Now for the political facts," continued the senator as

he delved into the unmentionable. "South Carolina, like every southern state, is proud. I know we should be ashamed of hunger. I know as a public official I am late to this problem. But in South Carolina we are also practical. . . . As a governor I had to put first things first. There were many able-bodied standing around looking for jobs. So, industrial development plus state pride resulted in the public policy of covering up hunger. We didn't want the vice president of the plant in New York to know the burdens. . . .

"The second political fact is that hunger is nonpartisan, nonracial. South Carolina's hunger is both white and black.

"Another political fact that must be coped with is the constant rebuff—'jobs, not handouts.' Many poverty programs have aborted because the people will not tolerate 'giveaways' and this is the greatest thing in my mail, the outright rabidness and hostility on this particular score. . . . I know the need for jobs, but what I am talking about is outright hunger. The people I saw could not possibly work. They were old people, sick, invalids.

"Let me categorically state there is hunger in South Carolina," he emphasized. "I have seen it with my own eyes. Starving—that is too dreadful a term. But the result is the same. Those weakened and diseased from hunger are dying from the disease caused by hunger. Weakened and diseased, they become emotionally blind. Their burdens and ours compound and grow. The hunger and the burden of the poor can no longer be ignored."

Fritz Hollings had ventured publicly where no white South Carolina politician had ever dared tread—walking in broad daylight through the worst black and white poverty in his state, from the Little Mexico ghetto of

Charleston to rural Jasper and Beaufort counties where Dr. Donald Gatch treated the shameful diseases of the black poor.

The evolution of Fritz Hollings, from comfortable moderate to bold iconoclast, dated back to the earlier days of the politics of hunger. As a candidate for reelection to the Senate in early 1968, Hollings had pleaded with Senator Robert Kennedy not to hold scheduled hunger hearings in South Carolina.

"It would ruin me," begged Hollings, insisting that in the race-poisoned atmosphere "hunger" would be forgotten and the only issue would be "Kennedy." Hollings needed both the black and the white vote, and the hunger issue might well destroy the delicate political tightrope he tried to walk. Kennedy relented and went instead to Kentucky, a state with two Republican senators from whom he felt no need to clear a political visa. Public attention thus focused on hunger in Kentucky rather than in South Carolina (as in the previous year it had centered in Mississippi instead of in Alabama) because of political considerations, and Fritz Hollings was reelected.

Kennedy, distracted from the hunger campaign by his run for the Presidency, died without ever going to South Carolina. Fritz Hollings, a moderate politician with a strong sense of personal honor, made the trip for him in 1969.

For Hollings, the political timing was right to take action on the hunger issue. He had just won a six-year term in office, and the Nixon Administration in its first month did not offer the white South much hope of turning back the clock on civil rights.* If the South were

---

* Several months later, however, the Nixon administration began softening federal policy on civil rights issues such as school desegregation.

ever to face its problems of black poverty, hunger would provide the least controversial beginning, Hollings believed.

Appearing before the Senate Select Committee on Nutrition and Human Needs, Hollings' February 19, 1969, testimony had more impact than anything the predictably liberal Kennedy could have said. The presence of a Deep South senator eloquently exposing the hunger problem in his own back yard had an immediate, momentous effect on both the politics of hunger and the politics of ignorance.

No longer could a senator pick only politically "safe" places to campaign about human suffering, ignoring conditions in his own state. Committee Chairman George McGovern was sharply reminded that the long-forgotten Indians who live on the Pine Ridge Reservation of his own South Dakota are as desperate as the black poor in South Carolina. Senator Javits had to face hunger in the bleak, endless slums of Harlem. Most significantly, other southern senators began to follow Hollings' example: William Spong decided to look at the poor in his own state of Virginia—as did Herman Talmadge in Georgia and Marlow Cook in Kentucky, who admitted that he had overlooked hunger a few blocks from his office in Lexington. Returning from their own hunger tours, these men called for immediate food aid reform, and solid southern resistance finally began to crumble on at least one crucial issue in the lives of the South's black poor. Even Senator Strom Thurmond was forced to moderate his earlier pronouncement that "there always will be hunger."

The two-year effort to create a national issue now was starting to show cumulative results, even though the national elections of 1968 had altered the cast of characters. Not only did a new President and his Cabinet now examine the hunger issue, but the congressional focal point for new revelations and political demands in 1969 now centered in the Senate Select Committee on Nutrition and Human Needs. Created to release the food issue from the conservative, antiwelfare confines of the agriculture committees, the Select Committee aimed a constant congressional spotlight at hunger. Poverty Subcommittee Chairman Joseph Clark had been defeated in the Pennsylvania elections, his fellow crusader Robert Kennedy was dead, and in 1969 Senate leadership on the food aid reform was assumed by George McGovern, chairman of the new Select Committee.*

The 47-year-old McGovern provided unique qualities of leadership at a time when food reform efforts required a broader coalition of forces. Inheriting the mantle of Robert Kennedy as a brief 1968 Presidential candidate, the South Dakota Democrat was gaining a national reputation. Although he lacked Kennedy's following and his automatic publicity, he also lacked the disadvantages of Clark's brittle, doctrinaire liberalism, and he brought new attributes to the job. He had worked on the food issue before, as President John F. Kennedy's director for Food for Peace; he was a farm-state member of the Agriculture Committee, which controls food aid; and he was a polite, low-key former college professor who could hold a committee together on a controversial subject. Finally, he had the services of William C. Smith, Congress's most skilled practitioner of the new politics of hunger.

* Other members of the committee were Senators Allen Ellender, D., La.; Herman Talmadge, D., Ga.; Marlow Cook, R., Ky.; Robert Dole, R., Kan.; Ralph Yarborough, D., Tex.; Claiborne Pell, D., R.I.; Edward Kennedy, D., Mass.; Jacob Javits, R., N.Y.; Peter Dominick, R., Colo.; Philip Hart, D., Mich.; Walter Mondale, D., Minn., and Charles Percy, R., Ill.

As counsel for Joseph Clark's Senate Poverty Subcommittee,* Smith had planned the original hunger hearings in 1967 and 1968. After the loss of both Clark and Kennedy, he moved to the new Senate Select Committee on Nutrition. Smith, 35, is a new-style social reformer whose goal is to make a practical contribution to American society. The product of an upper-class background and an impeccable eastern education, he practiced corporate law in his native Philadelphia, became bored with private practice, and decided to seek greater challenges for public service in Washington. Together, McGovern and Smith planned how to move the hunger issue forward in 1969. Their idea was to lay a broad base for food stamp reform by calling expert witnesses, such as anthropologist Margaret Mead, to make further field trips to areas of concentrated poverty throughout the country, and to escalate the issue with preliminary findings of the National Nutrition Survey. Smith and McGovern urged Dr. Schaefer not to wait the full year it would take to complete the ten-state survey before making his report, but to present preliminary findings from the first four states in January 1969. They believed that an early report might intensify the politics of hunger, which it did.

On the same day that Senator Hollings brought new honesty to the discussion of American poverty, McGovern scored a first victory and overturned a conservative attempt to curtail his committee's activities. The Rules Committee, dominated by southern Democrats and midwest Republicans, tried to slash the Select Committee's funds by nearly 100 percent in an effort to limit the committee's travels and outside studies. McGovern and Smith turned the Rules Committee action into a political gain.

* Senator Gaylord Nelson succeeded Clark as the subcommittee's chairman in 1969.

Seizing advantage of this potential defeat, they decided to dramatize the hunger issue further by focusing public attention on the negative congressional forces opposed to food aid reform.

McGovern and Javits carried an appeal to the Senate floor, challenging the powerful conservative establishment that has always dictated the Senate's rules.

"Forty percent was cut from our budget and it was cut in silence," said McGovern. "It was cut behind closed doors without any explanation, public or private. I can only speculate on the reasons. It is embarrassing for those who have so diligently worked to mold our farm and food policies to find that, in this land of agricultural abundance, many have not shared in this abundance."

For the first time within memory, the Senate overruled its Rules Committee. A clear majority of the Senate now favored facing the hunger issue squarely.

Together, Senators McGovern and Hollings marched to the new Secretary of Agriculture to seek emergency aid for the hungry poor of Beaufort and Jasper counties, South Carolina. Breaking Orville Freeman's rigid precedent, Secretary Clifford Hardin responded immediately, offering a pilot program of free food stamps to the poorest South Carolinians. And he made this emergency commitment without checking his decision with President Nixon *or* with Jamie Whitten.

The Hollings-McGovern visit to Hardin in behalf of the poor in South Carolina echoed the Clark-Kennedy Mississippi efforts with Orville Freeman two years earlier. In 1969, however, hunger had become a stronger, more viable issue, and a crucial change in political relationships had taken place: A Republican now controlled the White House, but the Democrats still held a majority in Congress. Although Democrats Kennedy, Clark, and

McGovern never had been close to Lyndon Johnson, during the previous Administration they often restrained their criticism of a Democratic President. Just as Republican Senator Javits and Representatives Quie and Goodell had a field day criticizing the inaction of Orville Freeman, the Democrats now had their chance. Now that Richard Nixon sat in the White House, partisan politics began to sharpen the Democratic food aid reformers' attacks.

Far more important than the political shifts, however, was an increased public and press awareness of the issue. Despite a conservative mood in the country, hunger finally had become a potent political subject. "Hunger is in, poverty is out," was the trite political appraisal. No one knew how long the issue would hold public attention, but the politics of hunger were moving swiftly.

Two years earlier, Hardin's free-stamps-for-South Carolina proposal might have been greeted enthusiastically by Kennedy and Clark when they were first learning about defects in the food programs. In 1969, however the reformers now were far more sophisticated about food program faults. Committee counsel Bill Smith quickly pointed out to McGovern that Secretary Hardin's concession granting free stamps to families with less than $30 monthly income in the two South Carolina counties would help only 203 of 1,700 families with less than $1,000 annual income. McGovern quickly attacked the pilot free stamp plan as inadequate, as did a delegation of South Carolina poor who came to the Agriculture Department to blast the plan as a "token effort." The Republican Administration had taken an important, if only symbolic, step—yet criticism and pressure for reform were greater than ever.

In many respects, President Nixon faced the same limitations on innovative domestic programs that hindered

205

Lyndon Johnson a year earlier. Equally burdened with Vietnam, inflation, crime, and poverty, Nixon needed immediate congressional support for the renewal of Johnson's surtax. Despite these limitations, though, the new President and his Cabinet had the advantage of a fresh look at old problems and programs, plus an absence of years-old commitments to the southern Democrats who dominated the Agriculture Department.

Secretary of Agriculture Clifford Hardin, an agricultural economist who had long been interested in the world hunger problem, came to office with the certain knowledge that he would face political ruin if he could not improve Orville Freeman's record on food aid reform. In addition, many influential members of the agribusiness establishment now privately urged the new Agriculture Secretary to push for bigger food aid programs and to resist efforts to take the programs away from his department. Leaders of the National Cotton Council and other farm groups knew that congressional support for farm programs was approaching an all-time low, as urban congressmen increasingly resented huge subsidy payments to wealthy farmers from the same budget as the stingy programs of food aid to the poor. The farm bloc lobbyists also realized that a Republican administration would show less enthusiasm for costly programs limiting freedom in the marketplace. As a result, most farm lobbyists urged Hardin to keep the food programs, which hopefully could be bartered on the floors of Congress for continued farm price supports.* The farm lobbyists and farm-state

---

* The American Farm Bureau Federation took a directly opposite viewpoint. The Farm Bureau wanted to kill the present farm price support programs. It recognized that farm program supporters won liberal votes by trading with the liberals for food stamp program expansion. Therefore, Farm Bureau President

senators like Herman Talmadge of Georgia decided to move forward on food aid, to avoid losing their political control if the programs were transferred to the Department of Health, Education, and Welfare. Thus House Agriculture Committee Chairman Poage combined food aid reform with the farm bill, telling liberals that the price of more food for the poor was continued subsidies for the farmer.

These farm lobbyists were following the same political script by which urban liberals had won food stamp program victories in 1964, 1967, and 1968. Whereas the reformers had threatened to decimate farm bills if food aid failed to pass Congress, now the farm business leaders and their congressional supporters planned to hang onto subsidies by threatening, then making a deal with food aid advocates.

Following the unusually revealing advice of Senator Allen Ellender, citizen lobbyist Choate also played this game in 1969, encouraging attacks on the farm subsidies and supporting plans to limit farm support payments to $20,000 per farmer. The wily old Agriculture Committee chairman had told Choate: "The best way to get those food stamps is to threaten the farm program!" Ironically, after the new politics of moral concern had created a national issue of hunger, the old politics of congressional vote-trading sought to capture and capitalize on the issue.

Secretary Hardin, therefore, warily declined when Robert Finch, the pragmatic, ambitious new Secretary of Health, Education, and Welfare quickly offered a joint meeting of their staffs to get right into the hunger problem. Finch, the attractive former lieutenant governor of

---

Charles Shuman frankly admitted that he wanted food stamps transferred to HEW, where agriculture committees would not be in control to make the trade.

California, nevertheless became an important ally for Hardin as lines were drawn within the Administration on food aid reform and other domestic welfare issues. A Nixon confidant for many years, the new HEW Secretary saw hunger as a political and social problem which could be dealt with rapidly and dramatically.

The entire new alliance between Health, Education, and Welfare and Agriculture hinged on a close friendship between two new appointees in the two departments. HEW Undersecretary John Veneman, a California Republican ally of Finch, and Richard Lyng, the new Agriculture Department Assistant Secretary for Consumer and Marketing Services, had worked together for years in California politics. Joining forces on the food issue, the two men brought Hardin and Finch together in a coalition that eased the traditional suspicion and hostility between the two departments of government. By the first of March, Lyng and Veneman were ready to advance a food program, and Daniel Patrick Moynihan provided the mechanism with which to do it.

Social scientist Moynihan served as director of the Urban Affairs Council, established by President Nixon to bring together cabinet officers concerned with the nation's urban and poverty problems. In setting up the council for the President, Moynihan created nine working committees, including one on welfare, headed by Finch, and another on nutrition, headed by Hardin. Staff groups from both committees began working jointly on hunger, with the White House staff work directed by 22-year-old Christopher DeMuth, a fast-learning Moynihan aide. On March 17 the two committees took to the White House a $1 billion reform of the food stamp programs, designed to lower the cost of food stamps and provide the poor with more food. Presenting the plan to President Nixon,

Clifford Hardin discovered conflicting motives in the politics of hunger.

"The most troublesome question is, how wide is the hunger problem in fact?" asked the President.

Replied Hardin, "We know there are six million persons in families with less than $300 per capita income, 25 million with less than $3,000 family income, and probably one half have nutritional problems, give or take one or two million. We're absolutely convinced this is a serious problem and one that with our abundance shouldn't be permitted to exist."

Nixon, somewhat skeptical but politically astute, then asked, "To what extent does our report reflect or respond to the Senate [McGovern] hearings? I've been on that side as a congressman or senator. Are we allowing their propaganda to pull us?"

"No," replied Hardin. "We've been very cold in our analysis. The absolute minimum a family of four can get by on is $100 a month for food."

"For $100 per month," quipped the President, "you can't even pay the interest on the bill at Gristede's [an expensive New York grocery chain]." When everyone in the room laughed, the President quickly became grave, shook his head in dismay at the disparity in living styles, and added, "You might see less a problem than the McGovern group. You might see more. All I hope is that we are really analyzing this for ourselves."

Finch, politically aggressive and action-oriented, quickly jumped in: "Let's take the play away from the McGovern committee and send a couple of your guys [White House aides] in a helicopter to Southern Virginia, for example."

"Good," replied the President. "Don't be props for McGovern."

Hardin also stressed political pressure. "I feel very much on the spot," he told Nixon.

"How soon do we have to move?" asked the President. "This week?"

"I have three speeches to give this week, the first one tomorrow night," answered Hardin. "And what I need to do when I speak is to say that I'm speaking within the policy of this Administration."

"You can say that this Administration will have the first complete, far-reaching attack on the problem of hunger in history," Nixon told the Secretary of Agriculture. "Use all the rhetoric, so long as it doesn't cost any money.* Now is the time to get right into it. Make a speech tomorrow night, and say you favor flexible price supports to pay for this. *Some* administration must grapple with the farm problem and limiting payments."

"This is specific, direct, and basic," Hardin said excitedly. "We can make this the showplace in the whole poverty area."

In his enthusiasm over Nixon's assent, Secretary Hardin missed two Presidential suggestions which bore directly on the problem of national priorities and would stall the hunger plan for weeks. Hardin thought Nixon had been joking when the President cautioned him not to spend any money. Two days later, Nixon's concern about the budget became extraordinarily clear as he angrily lectured his Cabinet for making only token cuts in their departmental budgets.

The Chief Executive also was not speaking lightly when he told Hardin to test the idea that food aid expansion might be funded by slicing into farm subsidy payments. This idea, supported by the Urban Affairs

* This quotation and all others at this meeting are reported as they appeared in the official White House minutes of the meeting.

Council and the Budget Bureau, had economic and political appeal to everyone except Hardin and his farm
constituency. Nixon was suggesting that, instead of ap-
peasing the arch-conservative farm committees to win
their support for liberalized food aid, Hardin take the
one action which would infuriate these congressional pro-
tectors of the wealthy farmer. Hardin simply pretended
he didn't hear the suggestion. Beneath his mild manner
and fixed smile, the new Agriculture Secretary is a shrewd
man who learned his politics as a college president dealing
with a state legislature.

The doubter at the March 17 meeting was Presidential
Counselor Arthur Burns, a conservative, 65-year-old professor of economics from Columbia University, who questioned why the poor could not grow gardens, wondered
whether the poor would buy proper food with food stamps,
and provided other hints that he soon would oppose action on the hunger issue. The President had listened to
Hardin and Finch's billion-dollar food stamp reform plan
without comment, and when the meeting ended, Arthur
Burns set out to kill the plan.

Immediately after leaving the meeting, Burns drafted
a memo to the President, criticizing Hardin's plan for
action. "There is serious question in my mind," Burns
wrote, "about the [nutrition] subcommittee's interpretation of Dr. Schaefer's evidence." * Aside from noting the
preliminary nature of the Schaefer survey, Burns stressed
every Schaefer statement that would attribute malnutrition to ignorance rather than to lack of money. (Staking
out a traditional conservative's position against granting
either food or money aid to anyone except the physically
handicapped, the aged, and dependent children, Dr.

* Preliminary results of the National Nutrition Survey.

211

Burns infuriated Dr. Schaefer with his interpretation.)
Pat Moynihan joined forces with Burns in downgrading
the hunger issue in a hurried memo to the President, expressing doubt as to whether there was in this country
any malnutrition serious enough to cause brain damage in
infants. Moynihan had in mind a reform of the entire
welfare system and didn't want to get bogged down on
the hunger problem.

Thus the first great battle over priorities was shaping
up within the Nixon administration. Dr. Burns, together
with Commerce Secretary Maurice Stans, led the forces
who argued that prime concern must be given to fighting
inflation by holding down the federal budget—a concern
that dominated the President's thinking as he concentrated on revising the Johnson Administration's 1970
budget.

The budget review followed a familiar pattern. Military
spending received only a cursory examination, and the
cuts which were made turned out to be illusory. As
always, the only real battle for priorities was among the
domestic departments (the departments of Agriculture,
Health, Education and Welfare, Housing and Urban Development, and Labor, not to mention the Office of Economic Opportunity) competing with each other for the
very limited dollars which had not been committed either
to the military or to old, established domestic programs.
Education was pitted against welfare, which competed
with mass transit, which vied with air pollution, which
competed with food programs, and so on. In short, the
most urgent domestic needs of the country were forced
to play against each other for money from the federal
treasury. As the politics of hunger developed in 1969, it
was becoming clear that the Nixon Administration, like
the previous one, lacked a mechanism to consider ration-

ally the full range of national priorities. When the $2.5 billion food plan went to the President on March 17, it was submitted without consideration of other priorities. These other needs soon distracted his attention and that of other officials from considering hunger.

A week after the food program was presented, the Administration's attention turned from food to welfare reform. At a joint meeting of the Hardin and Finch committees, the two sides forming within the Administration became sharply defined. The Finch and Moynihan groups now aggressively pushed for the beginnings of a guaranteed annual income, the Burns group strongly opposed it, Stans cautioned more study, and Hardin frantically tried to turn the group's attention back to food.

Finch and Moynihan began by presenting a uniform federal income maintenance plan for families, which initially would cost about $3.5 billion per year. Arthur Burns' aide Martin Anderson, a young Columbia University economics professor, immediately attacked the plan as "directly contrary to the President's public statements," as too costly at a time when the President was worried about the budget, as publicly unpopular, and as adding both cost and numbers to the welfare rolls when the President was concerned about such increases. The Republican party, he said, would favor proposals to reduce rather than increase both spending and the number of persons receiving welfare.

"The plan *is* costly," replied Moynihan, "but the costs are small compared to the Gross National Product and the problems of the people concerned. We are the only industrial democracy not to have a family allowance system."

Unless the Nixon Administration moved quickly, Moynihan urged, it would lose out politically. Either the Sen-

213

ate Labor and Public Welfare Committee * or a Lyndon Johnson-appointed income maintenance committee headed by rail executive Ben Heineman would take the lead. "The Labor and Welfare Committee will lock us in if we don't float a Presidential approach in the next three or four weeks," argued Moynihan in fighting for his favorite domestic plan. "If we wait until May 15, it will be the Heineman proposal or the Johnson proposal—not a Nixon initiative."

Breaking into the welfare proposal discussion, Agriculture Secretary Hardin said, "We can't wait on the food proposal. We need to go ahead. We need to maneuver so we don't sidetrack the food question."

Hardin had legitimate cause for concern. Allies Finch and Moynihan now were preoccupied in a battle against Burns and others to win the President's approval of a radical welfare reform plan. Although a modest food program might have fitted into their welfare proposal, they stopped pushing the food issue as such. Aside from preoccupation with their welfare struggle, Finch and Moynihan feared that a food proposal—expanded beyond their design—would preempt money and attention needed for welfare reform. "We are fighting for money and we don't want food to eat up all the bucks," explained a ranking Health, Education, and Welfare official.

The first weekend in April, the President went to Key Biscayne to make final decisions for reordered spending in the Johnson Administration's 1970 budget. The basic emphasis was on cutting the total budget by $4 billion.

* Welfare legislation in this category is under the jurisdiction of the Senate Finance Committee and House Ways and Means Committee. The Nixon administration finally presented its welfare revision plans in August, 1969, and almost dealt a crippling blow to food aid reform (see Chapter XII).

214

The hunger issue had no advocates at Key Biscayne that weekend; Moynihan was there, presenting his welfare proposals to the President. Food reform was ruled out as too costly.

The first hint to Agriculture Secretary Hardin that food aid improvements had been excluded from the nation's budget came at an Urban Affairs Council subcommittee meeting. Hardin again brought up the food issue, and Arthur Burns said flatly that there was no money for it.

"That's not my understanding," Hardin argued.

"Well, that's the way it is," shrugged Burns.

Although they had been preoccupied for several weeks with welfare reforms, Finch and assistant HEW Secretary Lewis Butler made a last-minute effort to head off what they feared would be certain political disaster. With clues supplied by a former Johnson Administration official, the HEW team pointed out to White House counsel John Ehrlichman several soft spots in the Agriculture Department budget which could give way for food aid money. Ehrlichman then startled Finch and Butler by responding casually that perhaps the food programs should be transferred to the Office of Economic Opportunity, or at least that OEO should be given a major role in directing them.

The surprised officials had not realized that President Nixon now looked at the hunger issue in terms of his efforts to hire a new Economic Opportunities director. Without knowing much about the food problem, Nixon's aide Ehrlichman already had offered Representative Donald Rumsfeld a major role in the popular hunger issue as an inducement to take the post.

Finch's visit to Ehrlichman, however, failed to budge the White House. Equally unsuccessful were efforts of liberal Republican senators on the Senate Select Committee who sought a major Presidential commitment to the hunger problem. A few hours before the President's budget revisions were announced, committee member Jacob Javits met with Nixon to warn the President that he would be misunderstood politically if he failed to take dramatic action to help the hungry poor. "You won't be satisfied with the dollars, but you'll like the ideas," Nixon assured him. An hour later, a bitterly disappointed Javits read the President's budget message. It provided only $15 million above the Johnson food budget, with this money scheduled to be spent on salaries for nutrition aides. All the appeals had failed, and on April 15 it looked as if hunger were not in the President's plan for 1969.

Although Richard Nixon attempted to map out his spending and legislative priorities in a careful 75-day review after taking office, he underestimated the intense political pressure being built by the McGovern committee and the Schaefer surveys. As further National Nutrition Survey results started emerging in New York, both Republican Governor Nelson Rockefeller and Mayor John Lindsay called for substantial food aid programs. Fifteen governors now asked that their states be added to the planned nutrition study, clearly showing that they were more interested in finding the facts in their own states than they were afraid of adverse publicity.

Further pressure for reform came from the National Council on Hunger and Malnutrition, which sought to follow up the work done earlier by the Citizens' Board of Inquiry. Led by nutritionist Jean Mayer, the National Council's efforts ranged from lobbying in Congress, to developing grass roots support in communities throughout the country, to filing law suits in behalf of the poor. Acting together with the Columbia Center on Social Welfare Policy and Law, the National Council attempted court action to force the Agriculture Department to spend idle funds for food aid. The law suit increased the Nixon Administration's political sensitivity to the food issue as did the public reports by executive director John R. Kramer, who pointed up every sign of Administration inaction.

Senator McGovern, attuned to those Americans dissatisfied with Vietnam, huge military spending, and failure of the country to treat seriously its most urgent domestic needs, hammered away at every rumored or tentative food plan being considered privately within the Administration. Speaking graphically in terms of national priorities, McGovern always associated hunger with a broader question of national purpose. "Our President wants to lavish $7 billion to protect the missile sites with dubious military hardware," McGovern told the Senate, beginning an analogy which would be repeated often in 1969. "We can purchase with half that an end to hunger in America. I am at a loss to understand a sense of priorities which places a highly questionable antiballistic missile system above the needs of our poorest children for food which can turn them from anemic, often brain-damaged victims of malnutrition into productive American citizens. I am aware that the security of our nation must be the first responsibility of government. But after years of rising welfare costs, urban decay, and rebellion in our cities, I can think of nothing which would add more to the security of our nation than an immediate attack on conditions which have created these problems."

McGovern's political attacks increased sensitivity at the Department of Agriculture. Urged on by Californian Richard Lyng, who learned of an opening in the agenda, Secretary Hardin pressed the food issue again at an April 21 meeting of the Urban Affairs Council. His plea was the same. The pressure was on, Hardin said, as he now had to testify before the House Agriculture Committee. This time, President Nixon was impressed sufficiently by Hardin's entreaties to ask him into his office afterward for a long, private conversation. He advised the Secretary to seek more time from Congress.

Five days later, Hardin again pressed for action. At another Urban Affairs Council meeting at the White House, he cited a news story that morning which accurately detailed the Administration's decision against a major hunger program commitment in the 1970 budget.

"The hunger program is on the shelf," the Washington *Post* quoted an anonymous "senior White House official" who sounded like Arthur Burns. "There may be malnutrition in America, but real hunger on a substantial scale— I don't believe it." This anonymous official said the Schaefer survey was too limited to be convincing. (In Burns' view of priorities, inadequate food among the poor became a first priority only after he saw conclusive proof that millions were very hungry; serious malnutrition apparently was not enough cause for action now.)

"What should I say when I'm asked about the *Post* story?" Hardin asked the Council.

"We don't know" was the collective answer of the group.

"I'm all for you," said Budget Director Robert Mayo, "but *you'll* have to find the money."

Moynihan and the top Health, Education, and Welfare officials now pushed Hardin to find the money for food aid by transferring it from farm subsidy programs, but Hardin realistically contended that to do so would be political suicide. Besides, the President had promised him the money, he insisted.

Again, the Nixon Cabinet faced the matter of national

priorities. Each of the other Cabinet officers believed that he needed to protect his own program ideas and to fight for the pittance of new domestic funds. If Hardin wanted to move on the hunger issue, he would have to reorder spending within his own departmental budget.

Adding to the outside pressure, Senator McGovern introduced his own national food stamp plan on April 29, at the same time criticizing President Nixon for making false promises to fight hunger. New York Senator Javits, his patience exhausted by still another Democratic move, went to the Senate floor to criticize openly his Republican administration. If the White House didn't want to act, Javits asked that it at least postpone a final decision until Republicans on the Select Committee presented legislation.

"Should there be advisers to the President who feel that the problem is not as urgent and crucial as I describe," Javits said, "then I would hope they would go out into the field as I have done to see the widespread and appalling conditions of hunger that demand much more comprehensive measures involving much greater expenditures than they [the White House] now seem to have in mind."

Javits and McGovern did continue to go into the field, first to Florida where they revealed callous disregard by state and county officials for the welfare of hungry migrant farm workers. Collier County officials refused to allow any food program for the 23,000 migrants whom they characterized as "federal people, not our people." The migrant children suffered from a lack of Vitamin C, as their parents could not afford to buy orange juice which came from the rich citrus crop they harvested. Local attitudes were symbolized by Florida Congressman Paul Rogers, who followed the tour in a pale blue

Lincoln Continental, bearing on the license plate a sign that announced "I fight poverty. I work."

The Select Committee then took a Washington, D.C., ghetto tour in which Senator Walter Mondale held a malnourished Negro infant in his arms on the same day the President, a few blocks away, sent Congress his budget revisions—minus any increase for food programs.

Javits and McGovern had invited Finch and Hardin to accompany them in an effort to involve the Nixon Administration in the issue, but Nixon Administration officials, in typical Washington fashion, had declined to look firsthand at the problem of hunger, despite the urging of Secretary Finch. At another Urban Affairs Council meeting on food and welfare issues, Finch asked, "What about moving on the McGovern trip to view the nutrition problem?"

Moynihan said he would check with the President, but doubted the wisdom of a field trip. Hardin then commented, "We know the problem is there. We can go along to humor them [the Select Committee] but I'm really against going on a field trip."

"If we don't go, it looks like we don't care," Finch protested.

Herbert Klein, Nixon's Director of Communications, publicly criticized McGovern for "traipsing around the country with television cameras" and said it was disgraceful for McGovern and others "to make hunger a political cause." A study in depth was needed, Klein said, before solutions could be offered. Klein's protest was a tipoff that the new politics of hunger were succeeding and that the Nixon Administration was feeling the pressure for food aid reform.

Actually, poverty field trips had meant much more than colorful publicity for the traveling politicians and

220

a chance to mobilize public opinion. Whatever their original reasons, the Kennedys, McGoverns, Javitses and now new Senators like Marlow Cook of Kentucky changed their attitudes and commitments after they descended from their airconditioned offices, bureaucratic statistics, and narrow Washington political perspective to smell the inside of a slum apartment or a migrant worker's shack. Their ideas on poverty became very personal after speaking to poor women who desperately wanted to care adequately for their children, but simply could not manage without government help. Even 78-year-old Senator Ellender mellowed considerably after going on the Florida hunger tour. He started out on the trip skeptical, with remarks that indicated callousness to human need, but the Ellender who returned to Washington became an advocate for better food aid programs.

Most Washington bureaucrats and congressmen remained blissfully unaware of the importance, especially in a time of social revolution from below, of listening to the poor articulate their own desires and their problems. "I was poor myself and know what it's like," or "it's all right here in the reports," were the defenses of Washington officials who declined to see firsthand how the "other America" was living and thinking. The Nixon Administration followed this traditional pattern; its principal concern on the issue centered on Washington politics.

Senator McGovern had carefully escalated his pressure on the Nixon Administration from the first day the new President took office. On May 1 McGovern tightened the screw one further turn, laying an obvious political trap: He publicly invited Secretaries Finch and Hardin to testify before the Senate Select Committee on May 5 and 6.

On hearing of the public invitations, Agriculture official Lyng placed an urgent call to Budget Director Mayo.

"Well, this is the moment of truth," said Lyng. "What are you going to do?"

Agriculture Secretary Hardin and Health, Education and Welfare Secretary Finch knew they had been placed in an untenable situation—that they faced a politcal roasting before the McGovern Committee. With McGovern in possession of virtually all the administration's confidential position papers on the food issue, Finch and Hardin knew they would be asked why their own proposals had not been implemented. Their appearance would be even more embarrassing after the Washington *Post* had published a front page story on May 3 describing the unapproved Hardin-Finch hunger plan in detail. Bill Smith had leaked the story to the *Post* to build further pressure for action. Hardin and Finch would now have to explain to the committee why their own program had not been approved.

Since the Administration's first days, the flow of public opinion fostered by responsible journalism and candid discussion among top Nixon officials contributed greatly to the pressure for action. From the beginning, the Nixon hunger proposals did not remain tightly held secrets like the Johnson Administration proposals—which might have been pressured into law if they had been known publicly in 1968. Nixon sought at the outset to contrast his "open administration" with Johnson's execessive secrecy. Officials in 1969 were less terrorized by Presidential temper than they had been a year earlier. Moynihan and Finch used the mechanism of the Urban Affairs Council and the news media to gain support for their battles within the administration. Finally, many Democratic holdovers remained in middle-echelon positions in the early days of the new Administration, offering a free flow of information to Democrats on Capitol Hill and to the press.

With the added pressure of the Washington *Post* story, old friends Lyng (from Agriculture) and Veneman (from Health, Education, and Welfare) met throughout the weekend in an effort to write testimony for their bosses and to plan some kind of defensive strategy. They had fought for a major food program and had not won one. What could they say when George McGovern and Walter Mondale asked what had happened to their food proposal? Veneman and Lyng built testimony emphasizing every possible advance they could think of in the war on hunger. But Sunday night they threw away their drafts and decided that their bosses should go back to the White House for another try at President Nixon.

Finch and Hardin met at 11 a.m. Monday, May 5, with Presidential Assistants Ehrlichman and Moynihan, again to seek approval of their food reform proposal, and to predict political disaster the following morning when they testified before the McGovern committee. Within two hours the President made a decision, one that was shaped largely by politics of circumstances.

"Tell Mayo to get the money," the President told his top aides, "and get it from someplace else than Agriculture."

After more than two years of battle, a President of the United States committed himself publicly to deal seriously with the problem of hunger in America. The President was asking for an additional $270 million for fiscal 1970, which would be raised to $1 billion for 1971. Now the task would be to translate a Presidential declaration into a reality of more food for the poor.

# CHAPTER XII

# Let Them Eat Promises

A DEDICATED GROUP OF MEN AND WOMEN HAD moved the nation's conscience; the President had promised "to end hunger in America for all time"; the Senate approved an emergency resolution increasing the food stamp authorization; and Annie White's family in Cleveland, Mississippi, still did not have enough to eat.

More than two years have passed since Senator Robert Kennedy's visit touched off a new politics of hunger in America, but little has changed in the lives of Annie White and her six children. The Whites live in a smaller, flimsy two-room shack; their other, much-publicized dwelling was demolished—for unexplained reasons— shortly after the senator's visit. But the Whites do have a little more food. As a result of her encounter with Kennedy, Mrs. White now receives a $79 monthly welfare check, and uses $32 of it to buy $80 worth of food stamps which keep her family in groceries for a little more than two weeks. (A family of seven should spend almost twice that amount to eat adequately, according to the Agriculture Department.) Still one of the "neglected Americans" at the very bottom of the socioeconomic scale, Mrs. White is just barely surviving. Her $32 food stamp payment, $24 rent, and $10 to $25 monthly utility bills leave precious few dollars for clothing, health care, or anything else. Her children still do not receive the free school lunches that a 23-year-old federal law promises to the poor.

The entire route from the broad avenues of Washington to the dirt path of Ethel Street in Cleveland is littered with unfulfilled promises, crushed hopes, and tarnished American dreams. The promises of America, as set forth in the Declaration of Independence, the Constitution and the Emancipation Proclamation, mean little to the poorest of the poor, whose lot has not substantially improved. Hopes for a better life, which carried waves of oppressed peoples toward this country, no longer buoy the spirits of Americans who for generations have been trapped in desperate poverty. When an Appalachian or Mississippi family migrates to the city today it goes with full knowledge of the rats and the tenement rents, and its only expectations are that the streets at least will not be paved with plantation cotton or company town coal.

The last 25 years alone are strewn with enough unfulfilled promises to break the hearts of the most God-trusting and patient of men. When President Harry S Truman signed the Full Employment Act of 1946, the federal government committed itself to maintaining conditions in which useful employment would be available for every able, willing American. Despite the great expectations of those who supported it, this law has little meaning today for several million chronically unemployed Americans

225

and six million others who labor full-time at poverty wages.

The 1949 Housing Act pledged "a decent home in a suitable living environment for every American family," yet 20 years later the original six-year authorization for 800,000 public housing units had not been reached—while the need had grown to six million units.

In his first hours in office, President John F. Kennedy signed an executive order "to expand and improve the program of food distribution throughout the United States," yet more than eight years later the food aid programs remain totally inadequate.

As he signed the Economic Opportunity Act in 1964, President Lyndon Johnson declared a War on Poverty and announced that "the days of the dole in our country are numbered." Sitting on the rickety front porch of Tom Fletcher's shack in Appalachian Kentucky, President Johnson sought to dramatize the targets of his domestic war. Five years later Tom Fletcher sits on the same front porch, still barely surviving, still untouched by the War on Poverty.

In the 1968 Housing and Urban Development Act, Congress specifically criticized itself for the 20-year broken promise on housing, but Congress and the White House already are hopelessly in default on the new promises.

Each of these programs has stated idealistic aims; each has been woefully underfinanced; each has been snarled in the administrative difficulties of delivering a service from Washington through many layers of government to a poor man out in America; each has underestimated the problems of dealing successfully with poverty and overestimated the national commitment to get the job done. Each law also has been accompanied by a great deal of

226

what must pass for either national innocence or insincerity.

The nation has deluded itself repeatedly by assuming that passing laws with noble preambles or issuing well-meaning Presidential proclamations has actually solved problems. The nation discovers a problem, debates it fiercely, declares finally its decision to solve the problem, and then rushes off to a new concern with the apparent belief that wishes are automatically self-fulfilling in American government. Such, sadly, is not the case and the hunger issue is but the latest illustration of this point.

At the moment that Nixon aide Daniel Patrick Moynihad read the President's hunger message to newsmen on May 6, 1969, ranking officials at the Department of Health, Education, and Welfare already were contriving to cut back on the President's promise "to expand the National Nutrition Survey to provide us with our first detailed description of the extent of hunger and malnutrition in this country."

Rather than expand the ten-state sample nutrition survey into all 50 states, hopefully mobilizing local medical and political concern as well as gaining new information, Dr. Joseph English planned to end the surveys. As director of HEW's Health Services and Mental Health Administration, English's idea of "expansion" involved sending 47 of his technicians (whose previous jobs had been eliminated) to work on nutrition with state and local officials. "The surveys are too expensive," said Dr. English. When he served as director of OEO health programs English had fought for food aid reforms. He now weighed the nation's and a new President's broad promises in terms of his own narrow problems in managing a huge and difficult bureaucracy.

When a Health, Education, and Welfare official ex-

227

pressed annoyance, pointing out that the President's directions had not been changed, Dr. English reassured him. "That's all right," he said, "we'll just say we've reached the end of 'phase one' and call our new plans the *expansion* into 'phase two.'"

The President's message also was weighed carefully against other problems as the Senate Agriculture Committee met privately the following day. With President Nixon now apparently committed to substantial action, Committee Chairman Ellender and other cotton-state senators decided they must quickly initiate legislation to protect their jurisdiction over the food issue and to negotiate a political trade of food aid in return for continued, unlimited farm subsidies. As the year wore on, Committee Chairmen Ellender and Poage tried endlessly to weave the two issues together in a political process that will continue annually as long as food aid legislation remains under the jurisdiction of congressional committees whose members have a client relationship with commercial agriculture and a distaste for liberalized welfare benefits.

A close examination of the Presidential message itself revealed limitations in its ability to fulfill promises. On the positive side, the message and a followup Administration bill attacked three major weaknesses in the food aid programs by pledging to: Provide poor families with more food stamps at less cost; establish national uniform eligibility requirements for participation in food aid programs so that some counties could no longer deny payments to persons in obvious need; and provide a food aid program in all counties, thus eliminating the discretion by which local officials in 440 counties continued to decline programs. The Presidential program also called for establishment of a Food and Nutrition Service, increased

228

emphasis on nutrition in various federal departments, and involvement of the nation's food manufacturers through a White House Conference on Food and Nutrition.

Limitations to Nixon's promise "to end hunger for all time in America" involved the amount of money committed and the quality of benefits offered to the poor. Initially, the President's food aid reforms would not become effective until the spring of 1970 at the earliest. The President indicated that he sought only $1.5 billion for the food stamp program in 1971, thus underestimating by almost 50 percent the needs projected by his own planners. Finally, the revised food stamp formula limited its promises even before its enactment.

The Delta Ministry, a civil rights, poverty organization representing the black poor of Mississippi, quickly labeled the Nixon food stamp formula "a cruel hoax which rules out most of the poor in Mississippi," and food aid reformers, led by Senator George McGovern, also challenged the liberalizations for not going far enough. The crucial determinants, once again, are the cost of food stamps to the poor and the amount of food they receive.

The President proposed that families with less than $30 monthly income receive stamps free, in contrast to McGovern's proposal that families with less than $80 monthly income receive free stamps. This one flick of a statistic could cause enormous consequences both in program participation and in cost, because 3.5 million Americans live on family incomes between $30 and $80 monthly. Whether or not stamps are free could be the determining factor in whether these desperately poor families join the program. By denying free stamps to the $30–80 monthly income families, the Nixon Administration would save $384 million. For participants with higher incomes the Nixon proposal set the maximum payment of 30 percent of income. In contrast, McGovern proposed maximum payment limitations of 15 and 25 percent of income for various income groups of the poor. Again, the question was whether food stamps were too costly. The Nixon program proposed that a family of four be supplied with $100 worth of food stamps every month, while McGovern called for a $120 stipend. The Agriculture Department estimates that $100 can purchase a minimally adequate diet from a grocery store but that $120 is a more reasonable figure of what it costs to maintain proper nutrition in 1969. In fact, the Agriculture Department itself expressed little confidence in its $100 monthly food plan: "Studies show that few families spending at the level of the economy plan [$100 monthly] can select foods that provide nutritionally adequate diets. The cost of this plan is not a reasonable measure of basic money needs for a good diet."

While the new food stamp formula was being worked out, Nixon's planners examined every detail, weighing benefits to the poor against program costs. The economizers won out. They had argued that most of the poor should pay 30 percent of income for food stamps, rather than the 25 percent recommended by the Urban Affairs Council planners. Far from fighting for a $120 monthly diet, Agriculture Secretary Clifford Hardin had his hands full winning the $100 benefits plan. Right through the final day of Presidential decision, the economizers tried to set program benefits for a family of four at $80 monthly, which is $20 less than the cost of what the Department of Agriculture calls an "emergency diet."

The Nixon program would cost $2.1 billion (he requested $1.5 billion) annually to provide benefits to 11 million poor, about one-half the estimated poverty population in 1969. On the other hand, the McGovern program would cost about $4 billion to feed 11 million poor and $6.5 billion for 22 million. In either case, these goals were a long way from fulfillment in 1969, when only 2.8 million poor participated in the food stamp plan at a federal cost of about $280 million and another 3.7 million shared in the free commodity distribution program. Implementation of either the Nixon proposal or the more ambitious McGovern program will require far-reaching action by Congress and the Administration in 1970 and 1971. The promise of food aid to the hungry poor will become a reality only if the White House and Congress follow through on this commitment far more meaningfully than on past promises.

From the White House all the way down to the county courthouse, politics already has blurred the new commitments. When it appeared that the Agriculture Department would not spend all its food stamp funds in fiscal 1969, Secretary Hardin and his subordinates worried far more about how to cover up the excess than about how to quickly commit the money so more poor could buy stamps.

Hundreds of school districts continue to flaunt the Agriculture Department's new regulations requiring that poor students be given free meals on a nondiscriminatory basis. Department officials, anxious not to offend state and local politicians, contend that they are powerless to make the schools comply with federal rules. State legislatures still refuse to appropriate their share of the cost of an adequate lunch program for poor children.

A hopeful sign from President Nixon, however, was his appointment of Dr. Jean Mayer as director of a White House Conference on Food, Nutrition, and Health. The conference, held in December 1969, was designed to provide a breakthrough in terms of new efforts, particularly from industry and the universities. One of the world's foremost nutrition experts, Harvard professor Mayer has combined scientific and social commitment in his work. An authority on both hunger and obesity, he also has worked for social reform in Boston anti-poverty programs and spearheaded the National Citizens Council on Malnutrition. Mayer, 48, possesses both charm and courage (demonstrated as a French resistance fighter in World War II), and he quickly found a need for those qualities in the White house job.

When the Senate Agriculture Committee defeated the Administration's free food stamp proposal, he was disturbed to learn that the White House congressional relations staff had not devoted any attention to the food stamp bill. "We're simply too busy with the ABM [anti-ballistic missile] and surtax fights," Mayer was told by Bryce Harlow, Assistant to the President for Congressional Relations. "We can only seek votes on so many issues." A professor, not a politician, Mayer was appalled at this limited conception of leadership. "I thought the Administration would want to appeal to people who had no interest in the ABM or the surtax, but were vitally concerned that action be taken against hunger," he replied. In his baptism by White House fire, the nutritionist learned how human concerns could be lost in the priorities of Washington politics.

As Mayer selected participants for the nutrition conference, political operatives in the White House exercised concern over patronage, in which satisfying Republican politicians held precedence over attracting the most qualified delegates to the December conference on nutrition. All of Mayer's appointees to the conference were screened in a traditional White House political exercise.

Senator John Tower (R., Tex.) or his staff sought to veto the appointment of Dr. William J. McGanity, a Texas physician, as vice-chairman of a conference panel because McGanity had been involved in liberal causes. The doctor was invited to the conference, as Dr. Mayer moved him to another spot not requiring political clearance. At another point, White House political aide John Dent sought to appoint Mayer's deputy from the political ranks, but Mayer refused.

Donald Rumsfeld, director of the Office of Economic Opportunity, the agency with legal responsibility to promote "maximum feasible participation of the poor," opposed inviting representatives of the poor to the conference, because he feared an embarrassing militant protest. In Rumsfeld's view, the black poor in America could be represented by Negro doctors or nurses.

The battle over who would participate soon shifted from partisan and poverty politics to the politics of food. Rival interest groups in every phase of nutrition, education, and industry competed to dominate the program. The loudest objections to the conference makeup came from representatives of the cattle feeding industry. Industry representatives and their congressmen demanded control over a panel on degenerative diseases. The cattle fatteners feared that this panel would come out with a strong warning that a diet high in cholesterol from saturated fats (like those in the prime steaks which come from fattened cattle) can contribute to heart and circulatory diseases. To insure "safe discussions," several panel leaders chose not to invite advocates for poor people or consumers.

Political pressures such as these, repeated thousands of times, cloud substantive issues and slowly erode hopes in America. Solemn promises to fulfill the ideals of

233

American social justice can also be wiped out in a single decision by uncomprehending or uncaring officials.

On August 8, 1969, President Nixon announced a welfare reform plan which in one stroke could have negated his own May 6 program to end hunger in America.

When the President announced his "family assistance program" in a nationwide television speech, he thought he had ended a six-month welfare reform battle within his Administration. The President's plan contained three innovative provisions which merited accolades from most social reformers: The federal government would guarantee a basic national minimum welfare payment ($1,600 annually for a family of four); families with unemployed fathers would become eligible for benefits; and the "working poor" would receive assistance. These liberalizing provisions meant that 12 million American poor could receive welfare aid for the first time, and that most welfare recipients in the South would benefit from a substantial rise in welfare payments.

The President's speech did not mention the future of food aid, but his followup message to Congress on August 11 revealed that his Administration planned to eliminate the food stamp program after the new welfare plan went into effect, hopefully by January of 1971.

Most food aid reformers agreed that money ideally should replace the food stamp system. The Nixon welfare proposal, however, did not offer adequate aid for a family to meet any of its basic needs. It guaranteed only $1,600 annually for a family of four. A minimum diet alone costs $1,200.

John Kramer, executive director of the National Council on Hunger and Malnutrition, quickly pointed out that elimination of the food stamp program would leave 83 percent of welfare recipients with less total aid than they now receive. Unless food stamps were retained or welfare benefits dramatically increased, Kramer predicted that the new Nixon program would end up as "a family deprivation system." While Kramer and Senators McGovern and Mondale attacked the proposal to eliminate food stamps, presidential adviser Jean Mayer publicly stated that the food stamp commitment would be kept, and began fighting privately to make his words come true. Mayer was certain that the President himself truly believed in his food commitment and would stand by it.

It quickly became apparent that President Nixon himself had not understood the very special role of the food stamp program in fulfilling his May 6 promise "to put an end to hunger in America itself for all time." The President had stated that all American families would be guaranteed the $1,200 annually needed (by a family of four) to purchase a minimum diet at a cost of no more than 30 percent of family income. The very poor would receive free the $1,200 worth of food stamps needed to buy the barest adequate diet. The President's May 6 proposal made a special commitment to help poor families meet only their food needs, not to eliminate their total poverty problem. If a family were willing to commit 25 or 30 percent of its meager funds to purchase an adequate diet, then the government would make up the rest of the cost of that diet. *No cash program could fulfill this same goal unless the program provided enough money so that families could purchase an adequate diet and still have enough money left over to meet other absolute necessities.* The Nixon welfare proposal provided less than one-half the funds needed to meet bare needs. Without the special features of the food stamp program, a family of four would need $4,000 annual income in order to purchase a minimum diet for no more than 30 percent of income.

The proposal to eliminate food stamps [finally reversed by liberal pressure] was recommended by Moynihan and his staff. Moynihan, the principal advocate of family security system, always had been opposed in theory to programs using special currency such as food stamps. From the beginning, he favored a cash welfare system that would eliminate the need for a special food program. Moynihan's plans went awry, however, when pressure from the McGovern committee forced action on the food issue in early May, before the Urban Affairs adviser gained approval of his welfare plan.

Even before the President had announced the May 6 food program, Moynihan and his staff had discovered that the food stamp program interfered with principal features of their family assistance program formula. Specifically, the extra money provided by food stamps snarled the formula's intended work incentive for the welfare poor. One solution to this dilemma would have been to raise welfare benefits enough to lift the poor out of poverty. But this solution was considered too costly, and politically, it was out of the question. Therefore, food stamps were eliminated from the welfare plan both to save money and to make the welfare formula work neatly.

In the view of close observers, the White House staff did not brazenly disregard food needs in the decision to drop the stamp program. Most likely, Moynihan and other Presidential aides never fully considered the meaning and consequences of a commitment to guarantee the poor at least a bare minimum diet for no more than 30 percent of their income; a commitment made by a nation that can boast of its average family spending only 17 percent of income for food.

The arithmetic of President Nixon's food proposal was clear, but it escaped the attention of his closest aides as their attention turned to other problems, other pressures, and other politics. In a government that has traditionally functioned at highest efficiency only at the level of political or national security crisis, the malnutrition of poor Americans seldom held the attention of the nation's top leadership for more than an instant. In just this manner has the nation for many years made commitments to its poor citizens and then forgotten or reneged on them. That this need not be the case, however, is evidenced by the success of other government ventures—where a national commitment to scientific progress produced atomic weaponry and placed men on the moon. There is no reason why this nation could not attack its domestic problems with the same determination, the same dedication.

If the nation is willing to make the commitment, a number of practical courses are available for immediate improvement of the nutritional health of the poor. These goals are readily achievable at the cost of several billion dollars annually if the nation becomes genuinely committed to achieving them:

*Reform of the food stamp program to supply adequate nutrition at minimum cost to all poor families.* A workable program should provide free food stamps to all families with less than $1,200 annual income and should charge no more than 20 percent of income to families with more income. (Even a 20 percent payment will require sacrifice of other needs by a family with less than $2,400 annual income.) Qualification for participation in the program should come automatically on filing of income tax returns or through a simple declaration of need. Food stamps should be mailed to participants or made available at post offices. Purchase should be permitted in varying amounts throughout the month, rather than the present requirements of a lump-sum payment either monthly or bimonthly. Barring a major income maintenance program which would lessen the need for food aid, an adequate food stamp program would cost initially a minimum of $3 or $4 billion annually.

*Improvement of the commodity distribution program by including low-cost, highly fortified foods and by adding other foods on the basis of nutritional needs.* Counties should be required to distribute all available food items to the needy. Although the commodity program is less efficient than food stamps, this program in 1969 served 3.7 million poor Americans in almost one-half the nation's counties. A switchover to the food stamp program should not be made abruptly until the stamp program is completely reformed to meet the needs of the poorest Americans.

*Expansion of the school lunch program to provide a highly nutritious lunch to every American school child.* The ultimate goal, achievable for about $4.5 billion total cost annually, should be a free lunch for every child. The immediate goals should be provision of free lunches to all poor children, extension of the program to schools without kitchens by use of private caterers and central kitchens, and improvement of the nutritional quality of lunches by the addition of fortified foods. The federal government should increase its financial support, require a state financial contribution, and enforce its own guidelines to insure that poor children receive free or reduced-price meals on a nondiscriminatory basis.

In addition, the federal government should:

*Require enrichment and fortification of basic food products such as milk and flour, and encourage the development and marketing of more low-cost, highly fortified foods.* It should insist that industry provide simplified labels spelling out the contents of food products by nutrient in percentage terms. For example, the label on every can of baby food or package of frankfurters should specify the percentage of protein, fat, starch, sugar, etc., in the product, as well as the vitamin and mineral content.

*Support nutrition education classes in elementary and secondary schools and encourage nutrition education efforts by such organizations as the Advertising Council of America, and other private approaches to mass media.*

*Provide nutritional supplements to pregnant and nursing mothers and to infants in the poverty population, preferably through neighborhood health centers.* These supplements should be prescribed medically and provided as part of health care services.

*Expand the program of federally assisted neighborhood health centers to provide medical care in all urban and rural poverty areas.*

*Improve the availability of free family planning services in poverty neighborhoods.*

*Expand federal sewer and water grant programs to low-income rural communities and require that services from such grants be made available to all residents.*

*Expand the National Nutrition Survey to all 50 states, and then continue monitoring nutritional health data by development of a reporting system through federal, state, and county public health services.*

*Support training of more skilled persons in related fields of nutrition with concentration on medical educa-*

*tion, public health services, and institutional feeding,
and finally,*

*Transfer jurisdiction over federal food aid programs
from the Department of Agriculture and the agriculture
committees of Congress to the Department of Health,
Education, and Welfare and the congressional committees
concerned principally with human welfare problems.*

Judging from past experience with other social legislation, a full-fledged national commitment will require
a basic reorientation of attitudes concerning federal aid
to the poorest Americans. This nation has never decided
that its government should guarantee every citizen an
adequate diet. Food aid to the poor simply is not viewed
by affluent Americans in the same light as aid to other
segments of society—whether aid takes the form of crop
subsidy payments, oil depletion allowances, ship building subsidies, government-guaranteed home loans, or a
thousand other government benefits which touch various
groups of Americans. This strange inconsistency of attitudes about federal benefits was dramatized in 1969
by arch-reactionary Representative Otto Passman of
Louisiana, who told the House about attitudes in his
congressional district toward food aid reform. Angered
by discussion of more food aid to the poor, a constituent
wrote Passman "humorously" recommending that the
hungry poor would be better motivated to seek work and
grow gardens if their federal food aid consisted of Army
C rations placed in garbage dumps. The constituent concluded his letter by thanking Passman for "the wonderful
[government] benefits you have provided this area."

Ben W. Heineman, chairman of the President's Commission on Income Maintenance Programs,* described

240

this American attitude to the McGovern Committee: "It has been public policy to have the nonpoor decide what the poor need, and to provide them with these things rather than with money which could be misspent. It has generally been believed that dependency and poverty spring from faulty values, laziness, apathy, and the like, and the treatment of poor and dependent families should include rehabilitation, services, and guidance."

These attitudes are illustrated in high public office when an Agriculture Secretary (Orville Freeman) dismisses the idea of a cash assistance system for food aid on grounds that old people "would use the money to play bingo" or a Presidential counselor (Arthur Burns) worries that even food stamps are not a foolproof way of feeding the poor because "they may buy potato chips and soft drinks." Such scornful attitudes toward the unworthiness and lack of capability of the poor have led to policies of providing minimum survival aid only after the most careful restraints are placed on the poor man's freedom.

After visiting the poor in America, Heineman rejected these hostile characterizations of the poor. "Given the extremely low income of many of our [poor] witnesses," said Heineman, "I was amazed at how they could manage at all. They often displayed incredible ingenuity in food preparation and provided as much variety and as balanced a diet as could be expected. Ingenuity, however, cannot compensate for the lack of cash to buy meats, fruits, vegetables, and milk."

Heineman, chairman of the board of Northwest In-

* President Lyndon Johnson appointed this study group in 1968. It was scheduled to present its recommendations in late 1969.

dustries, and a man who has changed his own attitudes after studying welfare programs, concluded that "our current food programs are encroachments on individual freedom of choice."

As the politics of hunger gain momentum, it is natural that discussion should move toward broader issues of public welfare. If the poor are malnourished mainly because they lack money, then a more fundamental approach to their problems might be taken by radically revising the nation's patchwork welfare benefits or by providing a guaranteed annual income. From a practical standpoint, a food program provides only limited assistance if a family still lacks money for adequate clothing, housing, and medical care.

In a broader sense, one of the greatest handicaps for the poor is their total sense of powerlessness, their feeling of complete impotence within the cycle of poverty and dependency. These feelings are augmented by a welfare system in which the dole is grudgingly given and regimentally supervised. The use of food stamps in itself can be a degrading experience which leads proud men to go hungry rather than be marked out as helpless. When the poor person goes to the grocery store, federal regulations require that he hand the food stamp book to the grocer, who then removes the proper amount of stamps. The objective of this regulation is to discourage trading or selling of food stamps. If the poor man's pride already suffers, not being trusted to tear out his own stamps is just one further indignity.

At the heart of the matter is whether the poor are to be given their survival money in such paternalistic fashion that they are degraded as human beings and limited in exercise of the freedom essential to ending their dependency. For the poor black in Mississippi, for example,

242

the required relationship with a county welfare official often may be just as degrading as that with the plantation patron. "Dignity is very important," says Dr. Mayer. "Very poor Americans need to eat what other Americans eat so they feel they are a part of this country."

Of course old people will play bingo. Of course the poor will spend money foolishly or whimsically or indulgently, just as the middle class and the rich do. One cannot insure that the poor will spend money wisely any more than that the wealthy will use their multiple government subsidies wisely. The question is whether we in this country are willing to permit even the poorest, most unfortunate Americans the honor of not having to beg for existence, of not having to go through one line after another answering questions and identifying themselves as the poor who live at the will of the state. I would strongly argue that the poor in affluent America should be given this opportunity to succeed or fail, to feed their children or drink beer, to live more nearly as other Americans do.

The poorest Americans who have been buried in the Deep South, the Appalachian hills, the Indian reservations, the *barrios* of the Southwest, and the big city ghetto did not fail to make it in America simply because they lacked ambition or ability. The plantation system, the migrant system, the mining system, the Indian welfare system all created long odds against a man's breaking out of a cycle of abject, dependent peonage. On that basis alone, justice demands that every American be guaranteed a decent minimum income.

Arguments for a minimum income plan to replace present categorical aid programs can be advanced strictly in terms of cost effectiveness. The cost to America eventually should be less and the results better if men have enough money to fend for themselves. The public sector could devote its money more effectively toward job training and education than toward building an increasing bureaucratic structure to superintend welfare and food programs. The growth of even more patchwork programs seems inevitable as legislation is now introduced in Congress calling for a "clothing stamp" program.

"We ought not to be talking about giving people 'food stamps' or 'bed stamps' or 'rent stamps' at all, except as emergency and interim programs," said Yale Law School professor Edward Sparer, who served as a member of the Citizens' Board of Inquiry. "We ought to be talking about income and income maintenance programs."

Income maintenance advocate Heineman points to the history of the two-year struggle for food aid reform and suggests: "If we somehow solve the food problem, we must then solve the housing problem. If, after more hearings, new commissions, television documentaries, and renewed public indignation, we solve the housing problem, we will then have to solve the clothing problem and the medical problem and the transportation problem and so on and so on.

"It seems to me that we must recognize all of these problems for what they are—interrelated attributes of the lack of money income. Perhaps, if we do that, we can make a concerted attack on the basic problem, rather than take time-consuming, ineffcient, and unsure routes such as the one we have followed in the past. For that path has put us where we are today."

Nixon Urban Affairs chief Moynihan hoped that the family allowance system would be a major step toward survival with dignity for the poor. Most of the original food aid reformers, while agreeing in principle with Heineman and Moynihan, are seriously concerned that

244

the poor in America will continue to suffer hunger and malnutrition, if reasonable food aid reforms now are delayed any longer. The delay could continue for years while the country begins to debate the very broad and controversial subject of family allowances, income maintenance, minimum guaranteed income, or negative income tax. As Senator Walter Mondale told Heineman, "I don't want children to starve during the ten years it is going to take us to debate income maintenance."

A reformed food stamp program would be a form of income maintenance and could easily be converted into such a plan if and when the nation approves it.

The promise of solving the hunger and malnutrition problem in America will not be kept if it is given only the same priority as other national promises on jobs, housing, and poverty. It will take the kind of commitment with which the United States builds a weapon system on schedule or decides in 1961 to go to the moon before 1970, and then, at the cost of billions of dollars, does just that.

Before the nation makes this kind of commitment it will have to answer the kind of question Apollo 8 Astronaut Frank Borman posed after his trip into space. "When we looked back over the lunar horizon at the earth," he said, "I found that I could take my thumbnail and put it up and cover the earth. You begin to realize our planet is a very fragile, a very small and very delicate piece of granite in the midst of a black nothing. And the thing that so concerns you is how in the world can the human beings that produced this technical marvel—a really mechanical miracle—how can we do all that and yet in all recorded history not have been able in some way to live together in peace and harmony."

This is a time of crucial questioning in America, and

the answers we provide may determine the fate of a free American society. Seeing that government still fails to act, a Dr. Robert Coles questions: "Why must these children still go hungry, still be sick? Why do American children get born without the help of a doctor, and never see a doctor all their lives? It is awful, it is humiliating for all of us that these questions still have to be asked in a nation like this, the strongest, richest that ever was."

Perhaps these questions have to be asked because we have accepted too much at face value about ourselves; we have accepted too many assumptions about the essential benevolence of our institutions, without really analyzing how they really operate and how they affect all Americans.

The politics of hunger in America is a dismal story of human greed and callousness, of immorality sanctioned and aided by the government of the United States. But it is also a story that does provide hope that men can change things, that men do care about fulfilling this country's highest ideals and do care about their fellow human beings.

A few men and women forged at least the beginnings of a new politics of hunger. None of those food aid reformers are revolutionaries. None threatened to tear the country down if they could not change it. But all did threaten and continue to threaten the status quo of American institutions, and that kind of challenge is not popular with the institution rulers, whether in Washington, D.C., Washington County, Mississippi, or Washington state.

The institutions have malfunctioned badly when a few men in a few committees of Congress have held such outsized influence over food for the hungry poor. The institutions are functioning badly when the nation declines to challenge the power these few men exercise within their special preserves in the traditional system. The institutions need reshaping when a great department of government and a few congressional committees can conspire together for years to subordinate the needs of hungry people to the needs of commercial agriculture. The institutions need rethinking when "local control" in America has for years given some men the option of deciding whether other men will eat or go hungry.

Our basic American institutions are on trial, and as John Gardner of the Urban Coalition has said, these institutions are caught in a savage crossfire between men who love only their rigidities and other men whose hatred of their imperfections blinds them to the promise of a free society in America. Our institutions may well be destroyed, he said, unless they are capable of change to meet human needs more adequately.

Students, in particular, are questioning the priorities, the values, and the honesty of their leaders.

Through the looking glass of America, one can see why the students are discontent. We do have the food; we do have the institutions for education and health; but we have not possessed the will to eliminate man's oldest scourge. Our ethics have become perverted when it is considered more important to starve a man to make him earn, than it is to insure that he and his children maintain good health and a zest for living.

Does the hunger issue indicate the corruption of our society and provide insight into the magnitude of our misallocated values? Or else, does this issue—raised by questioning citizens—reveal the possibilities for men to change the institutions, to meet the moral imperatives of a better society? Now only revealed, far from being resolved, it stands as a challenge both to those who criticize and deplore, and to those who claim America's system still can handle its problems.

"Something very like the honor of American democracy is at issue," President Nixon has said.

This nation oftentimes has not lived up to the ideals of its democracy. The struggle for a newer world and more perfect institutions may well fail. One can hope, though, that the modern politics of hunger will not end before many Americans respond to the plea of Senator Robert F. Kennedy after he had seen the hungry children of America.

"Someone wrote a number of years ago," he said, "that 'perhaps we cannot prevent this world from being a world in which children are tortured, but we can reduce the number of tortured children. If we do not do this, who will do this?' * It seems to me it is our responsibility, all of us."

* Albert Camus.

# APPENDIX A

## ESSENTIAL NUTRIENTS

The following chart lists some major nutrients (vitamins, minerals, and protein) and their common food sources, and some effects of severe deficiency of these nutrients.

| NAME | GOOD SOURCES | EFFECTS OF SEVERE DEFICIENCY |
|---|---|---|
| Vitamin A | Fish liver oil, butter, eggs, yellow vegetables, milk | Night blindness, skin diseases, blindness |
| Vitamin D | Fish liver oil, eggs, fortified milk, liver, sunshine | Rickets |
| Ascorbic Acid (Vitamin C) | Fresh citrus fruits, potatoes, tomatoes | Scurvy |
| Thiamine (Vitamin B₁) | Whole grains, yeast, meat | Beriberi |

(cont.)

249

| Name | Good Sources | Effects of Severe Deficiency |
|---|---|---|
| Riboflavin (Vitamin $B_2$) | Whole grains, yeast, meat, milk | Various skin ailments, scars on corners of mouth, and cracked or swollen lips |
| Pyridoxin (Vitamin $B_6$) | Whole grains, yeast, meat | Convulsions in infants |
| Niacin (Nicotinic Acid) | Whole grains, yeast, meat | Pellagra |
| Iron | Liver, other meats, green vegetables, enriched cereals | Iron deficiency anemia |
| Calcium | Milk, cheese | Bone and teeth diseases |
| Protein | Meats, fish, eggs, milk, cheese, beans, nuts, cereals | Kwashiorkor |
| Iodine | Iodized salt, fish | Goiter |
| Calories (measurement of food energy) | Protein, carbohydrates, starches and sugars, fats | Marasmus (deficiency of calories) |

Source: Department of Health, Education and Welfare.

# APPENDIX B

## RESULTS OF THE NATIONAL NUTRITION SURVEY

The following tables show dietary deficiencies revealed in preliminary results from the National Nutrition Survey, directed by Dr. Arnold Schaefer of the U.S. Public Health Service. Data are based on clinical examinations of about 8,000 persons in Louisiana and Texas, about one-half of whom were from poverty income families. These data are preliminary and reflect only the first subsample of the total national survey. Nevertheless, the data gathered to date show alarming dietary deficiencies in the poverty population.

TABLE 1
Laboratory Findings
Percent of Population with Less Than Acceptable Levels
(All Age Groups)

| | |
|---|---|
| Vitamin A | 13% |
| Vitamin C | 16% |
| Hemoglobin | 15% |
| Plasma Protein | 16% |
| Serum Albumin | 17% |
| Urinary Riboflavin | 19% |
| Thiamine | 9% |

## TABLE 2
### Hemoglobin Levels
### Percent of Population with Less Than Acceptable Levels

| Age | |
|------|------|
| 0–5 | 34% |
| 6–9 | 15% |
| 10–15 | 12% |
| 16–59 | 8.8% |
| 60+ | 8.1% |

NOTE.—A low hemoglobin level indicates a person is a candidate for medical treatment for anemia.

## TABLE 3
### Serum Vitamin A Levels
### Percent of Population with Less Than Acceptable Levels

| Age (yr) | |
|------|------|
| 0–5 | 33% |
| 6–9 | 29% |
| 10–15 | 18% |
| 16–59 | 8.6% |
| 60+ | 3.8% |

NOTE.—Vitamin A affects vision.

## TABLE 4
### Serum C Levels
### Percent of Population with Less Than Acceptable Levels

| Age (yr.) | |
|------|------|
| 0–5 | 16% |
| 6–9 | 12% |
| 10–15 | 13% |
| 16–59 | 16% |
| 60 and over | 16% |

252

## Table 5

This table shows the mean average height for young American boys and for boys tested in preliminary findings of the National Nutrition Survey. The children of poverty were shorter at six months of age and the difference in height increased by age 6.

| Age in years | American Average Height for boys | National Nutrition Survey |
| --- | --- | --- |
| 0–1 year | 26.7 inches | 25.5 inches |
| 2–3 | 32.7 | 31.5 |
| 3–4 | 36.4 | 35.0 |
| 4–5 | 41.8 | 40.7 |
| 5–6 | 44.4 | 42.8 |

# APPENDIX C

## THE RELATION OF INCOME TO DIET

The following charts and graphs are taken from the U.S. Department of Agriculture's 1965 Food Consumption Survey made of 7,500 households. The survey was conducted by asking families about food purchased in the previous week. It is not based on medical examinations of persons. The results tend to show strongly that the quality of diet is directly dependent on income, that the poor make relatively good use of their limited food dollars, and that the affluent spend far more money on soft drinks, potato chips, and liquor than do the poor. The survey also indicates that nutritional adequacy of American diets has declined since 1955.

TABLE 1
Quality of Diets
1955-1965

| Year | Good | Fair | Poor |
|------|------|------|------|
| 1955 | 60%  | 25%  | 15%  |
| 1965 | 50%  | 29%  | 21%  |

NOTE: Diets rated good met recommended dietary allowances for seven essential nutrients. Diets rated "fair" had less than the recommended daily allowances for one or more nutrients but at least two-thirds of the recommended allowance. Diets rated "poor" contained less than two-thirds of the recommended daily allowance for one or more nutrients.

254

## DIFFERENCES BY INCOME
### 1965 Food Consumption Survey

Dietary adequacy, as measured by the percentage of household diets meeting the allowances for all seven nutrients, was related to income. At each successively higher level of income, a greater percentage of households had diets that met the allowances.

High income alone did not insure good diets. More than one-third of the households with incomes of $10,000 and over had diets that did not meet the allowances for one or more nutrients.

### TABLE 2

| Income level | Percent of diets below allowances for 1 or more nutrients | Average number of nutrients below allowances |
|---|---|---|
| Under $3,000 | 63% | 2.5 |
| $3,000-$4,999 | 57 | 2.2 |
| $5,000-$6,999 | 47 | 2.2 |
| $7,000-$9,999 | 44 | 2.0 |
| $10,000 and over | 37 | 1.9 |

As income increased the proportions of diets that were below the allowances declined less sharply for calcium and vitamin A value than for ascorbic acid.

### TABLE 3
Percent of diets below allowances for:

| Income level | Calcium | Vitamin A value | Ascorbic acid |
|---|---|---|---|
| Under $3,000 | 36% | 36% | 42% |
| $3,000-$4,999 | 35 | 26 | 33 |
| $5,000-$6,999 | 29 | 24 | 24 |
| $7,000-$9,999 | 26 | 20 | 20 |
| $10,000 and over | 24 | 18 | 12 |

255

## TABLE 4

### Dollars Spent Weekly by Families for Food

| Income | At Home | Away from Home | Total |
|---|---|---|---|
| Under $3,000 | $15 | $2 | $17 |
| $3,000-4,999 | 24 | 4 | 28 |
| $5,000-6,999 | 30 | 6 | 36 |
| $7,000-9,999 | 33 | 8 | 41 |
| $10,000-14,999 | 38 | 13 | 51 |
| $15,000 and over | 46 | 19 | 65 |

## TABLE 5

Nutrients furnished by a dollar's worth of food, households in the United States by income, spring 1965
Low-income households had greater returns in calories and nutrients per food dollar, on the average, than households with high incomes.

A dollar's worth of food provided:

| Income | Food Energy | Protein | Calcium | Vitamin A value | Ascorbic acid |
|---|---|---|---|---|---|
| | Cal. | G. | Mg. | I.U. | Mg. |
| Under $3,000 | 3,150 | 99 | 1,090 | 6,860 | 85 |
| $3,000 to $4,999 | 2,860 | 92 | 970 | 6,320 | 80 |
| $5,000 to $6,999 | 2,570 | 85 | 890 | 5,990 | 81 |
| $7,000 to $9,999 | 2,380 | 79 | 830 | 5,320 | 80 |
| $10,000 and over | 2,100 | 72 | 750 | 5,180 | 82 |

# TABLE 6

This table shows money value spent by households in one week on various food and beverage items. These results from the 1965 National Food Consumption Survey show that spending on sweets, potato chips, soft drinks, and whiskey is related directly to income.

| Income | Soft drinks | Alcoholic beverages | Potato chips | Ice cream |
|---|---|---|---|---|
| Under 1,000 | $ .25 | $ .11 | $.04 | $ .51 |
| 1,000-1,999 | .26 | .11 | .02 | .70 |
| 2,000-2,999 | .43 | .41 | .09 | 1.04 |
| 3,000-3,999 | .53 | .42 | .10 | 1.08 |
| 4,000-4,999 | .57 | .64 | .14 | 1.33 |
| 5,000-5,999 | .65 | .98 | .15 | 1.43 |
| 6,000-6,999 | .72 | 1.18 | .19 | 1.60 |
| 7,000-7,999 | .79 | 1.49 | .22 | 1.61 |
| 8,000-8,999 | .74 | 1.43 | .25 | 1.69 |
| 9,000-9,999 | .75 | 1.60 | .21 | 1.70 |
| 10,000-14,999 | .87 | 2.12 | .24 | 1.91 |
| 15,000 and over | 1.16 | 3.79 | .22 | 2.16 |

# APPENDIX D

## COSTS AND BENEFITS OF THE FOOD STAMP PROGRAM

The following four charts show how the food stamp program worked in 1969 for a family of four persons; how much they paid for the stamps, and the value of stamps they received to spend monthly for food. Chief complaints have been that the stamps cost too much and provide too little food assistance to the poor. The last chart shows Senator McGovern's proposal and one Nixon administration proposal for charging less and providing enough stamps so families could purchase a minimum diet.

### TABLE 1

The following table shows what a four-member family in any of the northern states * paid per month in 1969 to participate in the food stamp program, how many free or bonus stamps they received, and their total stamps.

258

| Monthly net income 4-person household: | *Purchase charge* | *Bonus stamps* | *Total stamps* |
|---|---|---|---|
| $0 to $19.99 | $2 | $58 | $60 |
| $20 to $29.99 | 6 | 54 | 60 |
| $30 to $39.99 | 10 | 52 | 62 |
| $40 to $40.99 | 14 | 48 | 62 |
| $50 to $59.99 | 20 | 44 | 64 |
| $60 to $69.99 | 26 | 40 | 66 |
| $70 to $79.99 | 32 | 38 | 70 |
| $80 to $89.99 | 36 | 36 | 72 |
| $90 to $99.99 | 40 | 36 | 76 |
| $100 to $109.99 | 44 | 34 | 78 |
| $110 to $119.99 | 48 | 34 | 82 |
| $120 to $139.99 | 52 | 32 | 84 |
| $140 to $159.99 | 56 | 30 | 86 |
| $160 to $179.99 | 60 | 28 | 88 |
| $180 to $199.99 | 64 | 26 | 90 |
| $200 to $219.99 | 68 | 24 | 92 |
| $220 to $239.99 | 72 | 24 | 96 |
| $240 to $269.99 | 76 | 24 | 100 |
| $270 to $299.99 | 80 | 24 | 104 |
| $300 to $329.99 | 84 | 24 | 108 |
| $330 to $359.99 | 88 | 24 | 112 |
| $360 to $389.99 | 92 | 24 | 116 |
| $390 to $419.99 | 96 | 24 | 120 |
| $420 to $449.99 | 100 | 24 | 124 |

* Used in all states except Alabama, Arkansas, Kentucky, Louisiana, Georgia, Mississippi, North Carolina, South Carolina, Tennessee, and Virginia.
Source: USDA.

## TABLE 2

This table shows what a four-member family paid and received in food stamps in 10 southern states.*

|  | MONTHLY | | |
| Monthly net income | Purchase charge | Bonus stamps | Total stamps |
| --- | --- | --- | --- |
| $0 to $29.99 | $2 | $56 | $58 |
| $30 to $39.99 | 8 | 50 | 58 |
| $40 to $49.99 | 12 | 48 | 60 |
| $50 to $59.99 | 18 | 42 | 60 |
| $60 to $69.99 | 24 | 38 | 62 |
| $70 to $79.99 | 30 | 34 | 64 |
| $80 to $89.99 | 36 | 32 | 68 |
| $90 to $109.99 | 40 | 30 | 70 |
| $110 to $129.99 | 44 | 26 | 70 |
| $130 to $149.99 | 48 | 24 | 72 |
| $150 to $169.99 | 52 | 22 | 74 |
| $170 to $189.99 | 56 | 22 | 78 |
| $190 to $209.99 | 60 | 20 | 80 |
| $210 to $229.99 | 64 | 18 | 82 |
| $230 to $249.99 | 68 | 18 | 86 |
| $250 to $279.99 | 72 | 18 | 90 |
| $280 to $309.99 | 76 | 18 | 94 |
| $310 to $339.99 | 80 | 18 | 98 |
| $340 to $369.99 | 84 | 18 | 102 |

* Alabama, Arkansas, Kentucky, Louisiana, Mississippi, North Carolina, Georgia, South Carolina, Tennessee, and Virginia.
Source: USDA.

## TABLE 3

Inadequacy of Food Stamp Allotments, Family of 4

The following tables show the percentage of a minimum diet provided by the food stamp program as it operated in 1969. Few families were in income categories which permitted them to receive a minimum diet.

| NORTHERN FAMILY<br>Monthly net income | Total value<br>of stamps<br>received | Percent of<br>marginal diet<br>stamps can<br>purchase * |
|---|---|---|
| $0 to $19.99 | $60 | 60% |
| $20 to $29.99 | 60 | 60 |
| $30 to $39.99 | 62 | 62 |
| $40 to $49.99 | 62 | 62 |
| $50 to $59.99 | 64 | 64 |
| $60 to $69.99 | 66 | 66 |
| $70 to 79.99 | 70 | 70 |
| $80 to $89.99 | 72 | 72 |
| $90 to $99.99 | 76 | 76 |
| $100 to $109.99 | 78 | 78 |
| $110 to $119.99 | 82 | 82 |
| $120 to $139.99 | 84 | 84 |
| $140 to $159.99 | 86 | 86 |
| $160 to $179.99 | 88 | 88 |
| $180 to $199.99 | 90 | 90 |
| $200 to $219.99 | 92 | 92 |
| $220 to $239.99 | 96 | 96 |
| $240 to $269.99 | 100 | 100 |
| $270 to 299.99 | 104 | 104 |
| $300 to $329.99 | 108 | 108 |
| $330 to $359.99 | 112 | 112 |
| $360 to $389.99 † | 116 | 116 |
| $390 to $419.99 † | 120 | 120 |
| $420 to $449.99 † | 124 | 124 |

* Based on national economy food plan cost of $99.90. Northern costs actually range up to $109.50.

† No state presently has eligibility standards that allow participation by persons in this income category.

| SOUTHERN FAMILY | Total value of stamps | Percent of marginal diet stamps can |
| Monthly net income | received | purchase * |
| --- | --- | --- |
| $0 to $29.99 | $58 | 64% |
| $30 to $39.99 | 58 | 64 |
| $40 to $49.99 | 60 | 66 |
| $50 to $59.99 | 60 | 66 |
| $60 to $69.99 | 62 | 68 |
| $70 to $79.99 | 64 | 70 |
| $80 to $89.99 | 68 | 75 |
| $90 to $109.99 | 70 | 77 |
| $110 to $129.99 | 70 | 77 |
| $130 to $149.99 | 72 | 79 |
| $150 to $169.99 | 74 | 81 |
| $170 to $189.99 | 78 | 86 |
| $190 to $209.99 | 80 | 88 |
| $210 to $229.99 | 82 | 90 |
| $230 to $249.99 † | 86 | 95 |
| $250 to $279.99 † | 90 | 99 |
| $280 to $309.99 † | 94 | 103 |
| $310 to $339.99 † | 98 | 108 |
| $340 to $369.99 † | 102 | 112 |

* Based on southern economy food plan cost of $91.

† No state presently has eligibility standards that allow participation by persons in this income category.

TABLE 4

The following table compares 1969 food stamp benefits with those reforms proposed by Senator McGovern and by some officials of the Nixon Administration. The reform proposals would result in a lower charge for food stamps and provision of enough stamps to purchase a minimum diet.

Present and Proposed Food Stamp Coupon Issuance Schedules, Family of 4

| Monthly income | CURRENT NORTHERN SCHEDULE | | ADMINISTRATION PROPOSAL | | McGOVERN PROPOSAL | |
|---|---|---|---|---|---|---|
| | Charge | Total allotment | Charge | Total allotment | Charge | Total allotment |
| 0 to $20 | $2 | $60 | 0 | $100 | 0 | $120 |
| $20 | 6 | 60 | 0 | 100 | 0 | 120 |
| $30 | 10 | 62 | 0 | 100 | 0 | 120 |
| $50 | 20 | 64 | $6 | 100 | 0 | 120 |
| $80 | 36 | 72 | 16 | 100 | $1 | 120 |
| $100 | 44 | 78 | 23 | 100 | 9 | 120 |
| $150 | 56 | 86 | 39 | 100 | 27 | 120 |
| $200 | 68 | 92 | 56 | 100 | 42 | 120 |
| $250 | 76 | 100 | 73 | 100 | 57 | 120 |
| $300 | 84 | 108 | 82 | 100 | 72 | 120 |
| $330 | 88 | 112 | 88 | 100 | 81 | 120 |

Source: "Food Stamp Program and Commodity Distribution," U.S. Senate Committee on Agriculture and Forestry hearings, May 22, 23, 26, and 27, 1969, p. 4.

# Index

Hamer, Fannie Lou, 16
Hardin, Clifford, 204-11, 213, 217-18, 230
Harlow, Bryce, 134, 232
Hart, Philip, 202n
Harvard Law School, 66n
Harvard University, 29, 108-9
Hatfield, Mark, 152
Haynes, Dr. M. Alfred, 14n, 109
Head Start programs, 5, 8-9, 15-16, 28, 72
Health, Education and Welfare, Department of, 77, 82, 108, 155, 198
    National Nutrition Survey, 34, 38, 84, 140, 195
Healy, Patrick, 57
Hearne, David, 107-8
Heineman, Ben W., 240-41, 245
Heinz Nutritional Research Laboratory, 139
Helstein, Ralph, 14n
Henderson, Dr. Vivian W., 14n, 105
Hewitt, Don, 82n
Hill, Lester, 5
H. J. Heinz Co., 139
Hilton, Dr. Charles B., 106
Holland, Spessard, 47, 56, 62, 68, 71, 90, 94
Hollings, Ernest F., 198-201
Hoover, Herbert, 49
House Appropriations Subcommittee on Agriculture, 15, 84-97, 111
House Education and Labor Committee, 125, 130, 132
Housing Act of 1949, 226
Housing and Urban Development Act (1968), 226-27
Huerta, Dolores, 14n
Huge, Harry, 14n, 100n, 107, 116
Hull, W. R., Jr., 88
Humphrey, Hubert, 174-76, 185-86, 194
Hunger
    background on, 20-30
    definition of, 35

discovery of, 1-19
effects of, 33, 36-41
food industry and, 128-46
reasons for, 103-26
"Hunger in America" (CBS documentary), 115, 135, 181, 182n
Hunger USA, 111-18, 153
Hutchings, I. J., 140

"Incaperina," 131
Institute for Defense Analysis (Science and Technology Division), 117-18
Interdepartmental Committee on Nutrition for National Defense, 108
International Milling Company, 131
Irving, Dr. George, 84-85
Ivory, Mrs. Lily, 107

Jackson, Andrew, 117
Jackson, Jesse, 166, 169
Javits, Jacob, 49n, 83, 84, 91, 191, 201, 202n, 205
    emergency food aid and, 70-71, 82
    food aid reform and, 204, 216, 219
    Poor People's Campaign and, 171
    Poverty Subcommittee hearings and, 3, 5-6
Johns Hopkins School of Hygiene and Public Health, 109-110
Johnson, Lady Bird, 185
Johnson, Luci, 185
Johnson, Lynda, 185
Johnson, Lyndon B., 6, 49, 52, 67, 194, 195, 241n
    buget problems of, 72, 77-81, 148-50
    Poor People's Campaign and, 157-62, 168, 174-91
    War on Poverty programs of, 6, 15, 92

*269*

270

Resurrection City, 166, 170, 174, 194
Reuther, Walter, 29
Robert B. Green Hospital, 106
Rockefeller, Nelson, 194, 216
Rockefeller Foundation, 111
Rogers, Paul, 219-20
Roosevelt, Franklin D., 18, 49
Rosenfield, Steven, 19
Rowan, Carl, 182n
Ruiz, Father Ralph, 116-17
Rumsfeld, Donald, 233
Rural Development Service, 92
Russell, Richard, 5, 58

"Saci," 131
Schaefer, Dr. Arnold, 85, 140-41, 195-97, 203
Scherle, William, 124-25
Schnittker, John, 71
    Poor People's Campaign and, 159, 174, 178
School lunches, see National School Lunch Program
Scrimshaw, Dr. Nevin, 109
Seabron, William, 62, 66
Senate Labor and Public Welfare Committee, 5, 214
Senate Select Committee on Nutrition and Human Needs, 35, 36n, 39, 139, 153, 191, 198, 202, 219-20
Senate Subcommittee on Employment, Manpower, and Poverty, 2-3, 5, 14, 17, 25, 48, 67, 71-72, 74, 103
Senn, Dr. Milton, 9n
Shaw, Buck, 98-99
Shipley, George, 88
Shriver, Sargent, 67-68, 72, 78-79, 94
Shuman, Charles, 207n
Silver, Dr. George, 85
Sloat, Jonathan, 127-28, 133, 135-36
Smith, Neal, 141
Smith, William C., 6, 18, 29, 67, 68, 151, 155, 202-3, 222

Solidarity Day, 173, 177
Sorenson, Phillip, 14n
Southern Christian Leadership Conference, 150, 163
Southern Regional Council, 8
Southwest Alabama Farmers Cooperative, 70
Sparer, Edward, 14n, 244
Special Milk Program
    commercial industry and, 48, 57-58
    function of, 45
Spong, William, 201
Stare, Dr. Frederick J., 109
Starvation, 36
    definition of, 35
    "planned," 34
State, Department of, 108
Stennis, John, 5, 16, 72-76, 81, 117
Stennis, Tom, 121
Stewart, John, 174
Stewart, William H., 104-5, 110
Stong, Benton, 152-53
Sullivan, Leonor, 48, 69, 176n
Swift and Company, 131

Talmadge, Herman, 201, 202n, 207
Taylor, Atley, 4
"Their Daily Bread," 151
Thomas J. Lipton, Inc., 129, 143
Thurmond, Strom, 21
Trillin, Calvin, 166
Truman, Harry S, 225

Undernutrition, definition of, 35
United Fund Organizations, 111
University Club (Washington), 133
Urban Affairs Council, 39, 208, 215
Urban Coalition, 247

Vanderbilt University, 107-8
VanDusen, Dr. Jean, 32
Variety Children's Hospital, 108
Veneman, John, 208, 223
"Vitasoy," 131

Walinsky, Adam, 17

271